Helping Hands

Helping Hands

An Introduction to Diagnostic Strategy and Clinical Reasoning

Caroline J Rodgers
MChem, DPhil, BMBCh, MRCP(2014), DRCOG, PGCertMedEd
ST3 GP Trainee, Cambridge VTS, Health Education East of England
Cambridgeshire, UK

Richard Harrington
BA(Hons), MBBS, MMed, FRCGP
Honorary Senior Clinical Lecturer, Nuffield Dept Primary Care Health Sciences,
University of Oxford
Associate Director Graduate-entry Medicine, University of Oxford
GP Partner, The Rycote Practice, Thame
Oxfordshire, UK

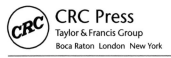
CRC Press
Taylor & Francis Group
Boca Raton London New York

CRC Press is an imprint of the
Taylor & Francis Group, an **informa** business

CRC Press
Taylor & Francis Group
6000 Broken Sound Parkway NW, Suite 300
Boca Raton, FL 33487-2742

© 2020 by Taylor & Francis Group, LLC
CRC Press is an imprint of Taylor & Francis Group, an Informa business

No claim to original U.S. Government works
Printed on acid-free paper

International Standard Book Number-13: 978-1-138-33082-5 (Paperback)
978-1-138-33086-3 (Hardback)

Visit the Taylor & Francis Web site at
http://www.taylorandfrancis.com

and the CRC Press Web site at
http://www.crcpress.com

To Chris, Samuel, Imogen and Margot.

CJR

Particular thanks to my wife Alison.

RH

Contents

Preface

We first met in 2006 when Caroline joined the Oxford Graduate-entry medical course of which Richard was the deputy director. The ethos of the Oxford course is to combine early patient contact with clinical problem seminars in an academic and evidence-based framework. We discovered that we had a mutual enthusiasm for visual learning, sparked by the use of patient videos in clinical problem seminars.

Various collaborations followed and were developed during Caroline's time as a GP registrar in Richard's practice. Caroline's interest in dermatology and her experience in devising an OSCE hands station led her to develop the idea of compiling photographs of patients' hands as a learning resource. A mutual interest in educational theory and clinical reasoning subsequently formed the genesis for *Helping Hands*.

We are very grateful to the patients (from Richard's practice) who kindly consented to be photographed by Caroline for the purposes of this book. They reflect the real work of primary care, combining as they do the commonplace and easily recognised with the rare and the complex. We hope that what follows will stimulate interest in the process of clinical reasoning in the context of the signs found on examination of our patients' hands.

Caroline J Rodgers
Richard Harrington

Acknowledgements

As well as all the patients who have kindly participated, we would particularly like to thank Professor Jeremy Taylor of Pembroke College, Oxford, for his encouragement in all matters relating to the graduate entry course and Dr Laurence Leaver of Green Templeton College for providing inspiration as a GP tutor and colleague.

Thanks are due to CRC Press, and in particular Joanna Koster, who took on the idea and gave us the opportunity to create this medical educational resource.

A number of colleagues, our expert reviewers, kindly evaluated the manuscript and their help is very greatly appreciated. We would like to thank Dr Antonia Lloyd Lavery (Consultant Dermatologist), Dr Lorraine O'Neill (Consultant Rheumatologist), Dr Tess McPherson (Consultant Dermatologist), Dr Ilana Levene (Paediatrics Registrar and Oxford GEC colleague), Dr Alex Murley (Neurology Registrar) and Dr Isabel Evans (GP) for their invaluable comments and guidance. Additionally, we are grateful to Dr Susan Burge (Consultant Dermatologist) and Dr Emily Adams (GP Registrar and Oxford GEC colleague) for helpful advice early on in the creation of the book.

Personal acknowledgements from Caroline Rodgers

Without the help of my parents (particularly my mum) and my parents-in-law, who provided childcare at key moments, this project could not have been completed. Finally, but not least, I wholeheartedly thank my husband Chris, who made me smile when the project seemed too much to have taken on and gave me his support, advice, encouragement and patience, which allowed me to finish the manuscript.

About the authors

Caroline Rodgers is a GP trainee who undertook graduate entry medical training in Oxford after completing a DPhil in chemistry. She has a broad range of writing experience including a highly cited (more than 200 citations) scientific review, two national prizes in communication (British Mycological Society Howard Eggin's Poster Prize and National Crystal Faraday Partnership Gordon Green Chemistry Essay Winner) and the publication of work relating to the development of e-learning resources that focus on diagnostic strategy. While a retained lecturer at Pembroke College, Caroline completed the Membership of the Royal College of Physicians and the Postgraduate Certificate in Medical Education through the University of Dundee. She enjoys teaching medical students and is currently researching learning styles and relationship with achievement of the graduate entry cohort.

As a doctor, Caroline has a strong interest in medical education and is particularly interested in how students and clinicians learn and teach the art and science of diagnosis. She has been involved in two published medical education projects.

Richard Harrington graduated from Exeter University with a BA in Drama and English prior to studying medicine. He has been a GP in Oxfordshire since 1990 and a tutor to Oxford medical students for most of that time. Since 2005 he has been deputy/associate director of the Oxford graduate-entry medicine course and has wide experience of teaching GP registrars and medical students in both hospital and community settings. He is a Fellow of the Royal College of General Practitioners and in 2017 was awarded a Masters in Medical Education from Dundee University for research based on Oxford students' attitudes towards careers in primary care, which has since been published. A lecturer at Pembroke College, Oxford, Richard is particularly interested in the use of patient videos in medical education.

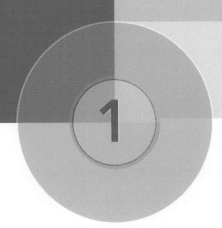

Introduction

1

'No teaching without a patient for a text.'[1]

Diagnostic strategy and clinical reasoning are not usually part of the formal curriculum at medical school. Currently, there are few resources available that introduce medical students and junior doctors to this area.

This book will help you understand clinical reasoning: the process by which a clinician formulates and refines an initial diagnosis with a view to developing an appropriate management plan. By being conscious of your approach to clinical reasoning, you will be better able to develop your clinical skills and diagnostic aptitude. You will also develop an understanding of why on occasion all clinicians are responsible for diagnostic errors – and you will learn strategies to avoid such mistakes.

As a medical student or junior doctor, this book will help you develop a critical self-awareness of the strategies you employ in assessing patients. The first section addresses strategies that can be used when taking a history, and the second strategies used when examining patients. To illustrate the latter with 'real life' examples, we start with scenarios based on examination of the hands, which is often the initial step in physical evaluation. A patient's hands can provide a wealth of information relevant to the diagnostic process. However, the strategies described are equally applicable to any part of the clinical examination.

This book will help you develop an understanding of the diagnostic approaches used by most experienced clinicians. By careful study of the illustrated cases, you will be encouraged to 'see' rather than just 'look' and to refine your powers of observation. In addition, we provide online resources that can be used for revision to help you learn topics in clinical medicine, and include a section on teaching clinical reasoning for medical educators.

The patients have been selected to demonstrate a spectrum of approaches used in clinical reasoning. They demonstrate the process of forming a diagnostic hypothesis including the intuitive *spot diagnosis* based on a single clinical cue, and more sophisticated *pattern recognition*. The more complex cases lead to a consideration of the various *refinement strategies* including *restricted rule out, pattern fit recognition* and *deliberate reasoning*.[2]

Whatever your stage of training, the following histories and illustrated key cases, combined with an introduction to the theory of clinical reasoning, will help advance your knowledge and clinical skills as well as develop a critical self-awareness of the diagnostic processes used by all clinicians. We hope you enjoy the clinical scenarios and learn from the process of studying them. We would like to thank the patients who kindly agreed to be photographed for the purposes of this book.

SUMMARY

- Examination of the hands is often the initial step in physical examination, and a wealth of information can be gleaned from the hands.
- This chapter introduces the main themes of the book – clinical reasoning, diagnostic strategy and bias leading to error.
- The structure of the book is described, which emphasises how strategies can be employed during history taking and examination.
- In addition, each chapter is accompanied by clinical cases that take a predominantly 'serial cue' approach.

REFERENCES

1 Bliss M, Osler W. *A Life in Medicine*. New York: Oxford University Press; 2007.
2 Heneghan C, Glasziou P, Thompson M, *et al*. Diagnostic strategies used in primary care. *BMJ* 2009;**338**:b946.

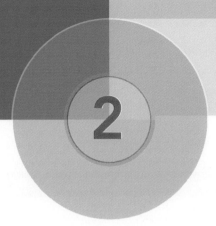

Clinical reasoning

2

WHY IT IS IMPORTANT TO STUDY CLINICAL REASONING

Clinical reasoning is in broad terms the cognitive process underpinning the diagnosis and management of patients.[1] Diagnosis can be viewed as the 'answer' that one arrives at after a process of reasoning, often seen as a 'diagnostic label'. Another important construct is to see diagnosis as a dynamic stepping stone and not an end point in the process of clinical reasoning.[2] Central to clinical reasoning is clinical decision making, which involves key critical thinking skills of:

- Hypothesis generation.
- Information processing and synthesis.
- Weighing up of evidence.
- Formulating a decision to be acted on.

Decision making uses a clinician's knowledge and powers of metacognition: the ability to reflect, reason and refine (**Figure 2.1**).[3]

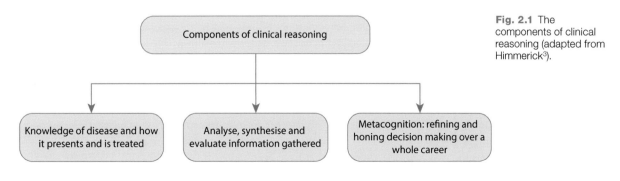

Fig. 2.1 The components of clinical reasoning (adapted from Himmerick[3]).

3

High-quality care and patient safety are the prime concerns for clinicians and patients alike. Optimal clinical decision making goes a very long way towards avoiding error (e.g. diagnostic failure or prescribing errors) and poor-quality care. Therefore, it is important that we try to understand the process of clinical reasoning and the ways in which we can improve it, rather than leaving it as a 'black box' (as clinical reasoning expert Croskerry phrases it).[4]

DIAGNOSTIC CLOSURE

It is important to recognise diagnosis as a shared process between health professionals and patients rather than the end point of the assimilation of information and pronouncement of 'an answer'. Knowing when to stop in the process of clinical decision making (diagnostic closure) is a skill in itself and also the subject of research.[5] When are we confident we have enough information to make a diagnosis? Do we need to request further tests or carry out a further examination? Also, it is important to remember that we should not accept without question the diagnostic closure of other clinicians if a patient's signs and symptoms do not quite add up. We can revisit the diagnostic process and observe how a situation progresses.[2] Sometimes we have to acknowledge that we cannot always apply a diagnostic label to a situation and that we are unable to account for and resolve a patient's complaint.

HOW DOCTORS THINK

Decision making is the bread and butter of a clinician's work on a daily basis. Yet this skill is often neglected in the curricula of medical schools worldwide and there is a call for better understanding and training in diagnostics.[6] There is a growing body of evidence to support the premise, that when diagnostic errors occur, it is often a failure not of knowledge but of the decision-making process.[7] We are beginning to build up a picture of the cognitive processes behind clinicians' clinical reasoning from research in both the laboratory and the clinical environment. With a better picture we can begin to develop and appraise strategies to improve reasoning and avoid error.

How clinicians might represent disease in their memories is under debate in the literature. Certainly, some representations are in the form of scenarios relating to previous patient encounters.[8] Hence it is thought that each individual clinician builds up their own memory bank of patient 'exemplars' (case memories), categorised in their memories and available to be recalled and compared against a newly presenting patient with similar features.[6] 'Illness scripts' are a second concept that integrate the information gained from clinical experience (exemplars) with knowledge (e.g. epidemiological, pharmacological, etc.).[6] According to Pellacia *et al.*, the construction of patterns in long-term memory (illness scripts) by exposure to multiple cases aids the development of intuition and hence non-analytic reasoning (NAR) (see below).[9]

DUAL PROCESS THEORY

In terms of models of clinical decision making, the most widely accepted is the dual process theory. It is generally accepted (with support from functional MRI studies) that, in making a diagnosis, medical students and expert clinicians use both analytic and non-analytic reasoning (the two cognitive processes that have been demonstrated to be both physiologically and anatomically distinct).[10–12] Use of a combination has been shown to have improved accuracy over a single approach.[13] This combined approach is known as 'dual process theory'; in this an intuitive (system 1) response (often using visual information and sometimes referred to as 'non-analytic reasoning') is combined with a rational and deliberative response (system 2 – analytic reasoning).[9] Qualitative studies exploring how clinicians make decisions have been carried out using dual process theory as a framework.[5]

It is important to emphasise that the two systems interact with each other such that system 2 can override system 1 thinking ('executive override'), and there is what has been referred to as a 'toggle function', meaning that clinicians can switch between the two systems during the reasoning process.[7] It is known that as clinicians progress from being novice to competent to expert, intuition and use of system 1 thinking becomes more prominent (**Figure 2.2**). But system 1 is more prone to error and mistakes made via this system more often go uncorrected since it is subconsciously employed.[7]

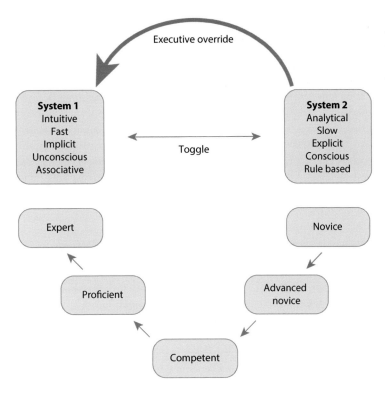

Fig. 2.2 Dual process theory.

COMPARING SYSTEM 1 THINKING AND SYSTEM 2 THINKING

As discussed above, system 1 thinking has been shown to be employed by both novices and experts, with a shift towards system 1 as the clinician becomes more experienced and has greater expertise.[13] However, there is a debate in the literature over the merits and shortcomings of the system 1 and system 2 approaches.[14] This tension stems from the reliance that system 1 thinking places on pattern recognition, and hence it may be more prone to error than system 2 (which is slower and more deliberate). Therefore, should we encourage the development of intuitive reasoning in medical education?

The use of system 1 in tandem with analytic reasoning has been shown to be very effective; examples include the ECG-based studies in medical students reported by Eva *et al.* and a study looking at dermatological diagnosis by medical students reported by Kulatunga-Moruzi *et al.*[13,15] Hence there is growing evidence to support the creation of an environment for the development of intuitive reasoning in the teaching of clinical reasoning. The extent to which medical students use and develop it is not well known, and since NAR is a skill that requires a great deal of experience of clinical cases to master, whether medical students should use it at all is a matter of debate. Thus analytic reasoning currently has the main emphasis in the teaching of clinical reasoning. Norman recently highlighted Croskerry's views:

> [Analytic reasoning] … can be seen as the superego of decision making, fighting off the primary impulsivity of [NAR] in favour of reality testing, analytic judgement, metacognition and affect tolerance. It is the 'conscience' of decision making.[10]

It is perhaps best to view system 1 and system 2 as complementary and not competing elements of the decision-making process, and if we are aware of the benefits and pitfalls of each system we can strive to maintain patient safety and quality of care in our decision making. We should perhaps raise awareness that, although extremely useful, system 1 thinking should not be relied on by novices and should be checked via an analytic system 2 approach. Reliance on system 1 may tempt clinicians to make errors via 'premature closure' (that is, a tendency to finish thinking of other possibilities once a primary diagnosis has been reached).[9,13] However, for the more experienced, since the time taken for arrival at a diagnosis is inversely related to accuracy, system 1 plays an important role in diagnosis as it often leads to a more rapid solution to a problem in the clinical context than does analytic reasoning.[11] However, analytic reasoning is not immune to error either; here errors are perhaps fuelled by a reliance on working memory.[10] This is explored further in the next chapter.

IMPROVING CLINICAL REASONING

A dual approach towards the improvement of clinical reasoning has been suggested which involves increasing the understanding and application of diagnostic strategy tools alongside the use of techniques to reduce error.[16]

Croskerry suggests that doctors can improve their decision making by gaining a better understanding of the ways in which it is biased.[7] Cognitive bias can be viewed as the flip side of system 1 thinking – a tendency to respond in predictable ways based on our past experience and cognitive patterns. Hence understanding and practicing 'cognitive debiasing' may make for better diagnosticians.[6] At present, this is an emerging field of research that is methodologically challenging, but a systematic review of available studies that involved interventions to improve analytical and non-analytical reasoning in clinicians has recently been published.[17]

Cognitive debiasing is not the primary focus of this book, but we include a section on diagnostic error in the next chapter and refer to possible strategies among the cases. Another complementary strategy is to introduce the concept of 'metacognition' (thinking about thinking – see above) into medical training, with the aim of improving decision making through increased awareness of how decisions are made. These strategies would hopefully run alongside a broad clinical experience, using every patient case as a learning opportunity.[6]

SUMMARY

- This chapter defines clinical reasoning and explains the importance of studying it, introducing clinical reasoning as comprising the key skills of hypothesis generation, information processing and synthesis, weighing up of evidence and formulation of a decision to be acted on.
- This chapter emphasises the aim of optimising the process of clinical reasoning in order to improve patient safety and quality of care, and avoid diagnostic error.
- Concepts in clinical decision making relating to 'how doctors think' are presented, and the representation of disease in the human memory (exemplars and illness scripts), as well as the dual process theory model in clinical decision making, are discussed.
- The pros and cons of system 1 and system 2 thinking are compared and the concepts of cognitive bias and cognitive debiasing are introduced.

REFERENCES

1　Linn A, Khaw C, Kildea H, Tonkin A. Clinical reasoning. A guide to improving teaching and practice. *Aust Fam Phys* 2012;**41**:18–20.
2　Ilgen JS, Eva KW, Regehr G. What's in a label? Is diagnosis the start or the end of clinical reasoning? *J Gen Intern Med* 2016;**31**:435–7.
3　Himmerick KA. How clinicians think: the evolution of clinical reasoning. *JAAPA* 2011;**24**:18.
4　Croskerry P. Our better angels and black boxes. *Emerg Med J* 2016;**33**:242.
5　Balla J, Heneghan C, Thompson M, Balla M. Clinical decision making in a high-risk primary care environment: a qualitative study in the UK. *BMJ Open* 2012;**2**:1–8.
6　Brush JE, Jr., Sherbino J, Norman GR. How expert clinicians intuitively recognize a medical diagnosis. *Am J Med* 2017;**130**:629–34.
7　Croskerry P, Singhal G, Mamede S. Cognitive debiasing 1: origins of bias and theory of debiasing. *BMJ Qual Saf* 2013;**22**:ii58–ii64.
8　Kassirer JP. Teaching clinical reasoning: case-based and coached. *Acad Med* 2010;**85**:1118–24.
9　Pelaccia T, Tardif J, Triby E, Charlin B. An analysis of clinical reasoning through a recent and comprehensive approach: the dual-process theory. *Med Educ Online* 2011;**16**:5890–8.
10　Norman GR, Eva KW. Diagnostic error and clinical reasoning. *Med Educ* 2010;**44**:94–100.
11　Norman G, Young M, Brooks L. Non-analytical models of clinical reasoning: the role of experience. *Med Educ* 2007;**41**:1140–5.
12　Kahneman D. *Thinking, Fast and Slow*. London: Penguin; 2011.
13　Kulatunga-Moruzi C, Brooks LR, Norman GR. Coordination of analytic and similarity-based processing strategies and expertise in dermatological diagnosis. *Teach Learn Med* 2001;**13**:110–16.
14　Croskerry P, Petrie DA, Reilly JB, Tait G. Deciding about fast and slow decisions. *Acad Med* 2014;**89**:197–200.
15　Eva KW, Hatala RM, LeBlanc VR, Brooks LR. Teaching from the clinical reasoning literature: combined reasoning strategies help novice diagnosticians overcome misleading information. *Med Educ* 2007;**41**:1152–8.
16　Gruppen LD. Clinical reasoning: defining it, teaching it, assessing it, studying it. *West J Emerg Med* 2017;**18**:4–7.
17　Lambe KA, Reilly G, Kelly BD, Curristan S. Dual-process cognitive interventions to enhance diagnostic reasoning: a systematic review. *BMJ Qual Saf* 2016;**25**:808.

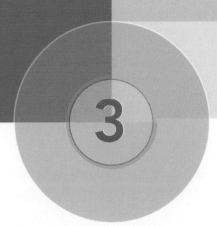

Diagnostic strategy

3

CLINICAL DECISION MAKING AND FACTORS THAT AFFECT IT

Career options for clinicians are diverse and require differing skills. Common to all is the need to make good decisions, but different specialties may rely on a different decision-making skill set. For example, visual specialties such as radiology, dermatology and pathology rely more heavily on visual pattern recognition and system 1-based thinking. Some specialties, such as emergency medicine and general practice, have a higher density of clinical decisions to be made in a short space of time.

There are numerous circumstances in which clinicians in different specialties are making important decisions (alone in a GP consulting room, in a busy overcrowded emergency department, as a team on a ward, in an outpatient clinic, at night in an out of hours service, etc.). We are human diagnosticians and hence a number of factors influence our decision making. These factors range from personal elements such as the clinician's mood, experience and level of sleep deprivation, to patient factors such as their willingness or ability to answer questions accurately and the patient's demographic, to environmental and system factors such as overcrowding in the emergency department and gaps in staff rosters.

For all clinicians, the question is, 'how can we optimise our decision making?' Which factors are under our control, and what changes can we make to what we do and how we function in our workplaces to help avoid error in the diagnostic process? This book focuses on raising awareness of the diagnostic strategies and tools we use to make clinical decisions, and briefly touches on cognitive bias in decision making and approaches to help prevent this (cognitive debiasing).

SELECTED STRATEGIES EMPLOYED BY CLINICIANS TO AID DECISION MAKING

Recent years have seen the publication of various studies into the diagnostic strategies employed by clinicians. Some studies have focused on the area of emergency medicine, in which there is a high density of decision making, and the nature of the strategies used by these clinicians is beginning to emerge.[1] Other studies have focused on primary care, out of hours services and junior doctors.[2–4] In addition, the point at which these strategies are employed in the diagnostic process is also being explored. For example, a clinical case may be framed using first impressions (such as the 'eyeball test') and initial cues, whereas checkpoint strategies such as red flags may be employed later.[3]

Heneghan *et al.* described the diagnostic process as comprising three stages: initiation, refinement and definition of final diagnosis.[2] His group attempted to identify the strategies used in each stage by primary care physicians. Different clinicians used different approaches to the same problem but some general themes emerged.

This book uses a series of cases to illustrate the following strategies:

- Spot diagnosis (used in the initiation phase).
- Pattern recognition trigger and pattern recognition fit (used in the initiation and refinement stages).
- Red and yellow flags (used in the initiation and refinement stages).
- Restricted rule-outs (used in the refinement phase).
- Probabilistic reasoning (used in the refinement stage).
- Test of time (used in the final diagnosis stage).
- Test of treatment (used in the final diagnosis stage).

ADDITIONAL STRATEGIES AND DIAGNOSTIC AIDS

KEEPING THINGS SIMPLE: OCKHAM AND SUTTON

William of Ockham (Occam) (c.1285–c.1349) stated a principle of parsimony that has become known as Ockham's razor and, in the context of a clinical problem, states that the most likely correct diagnosis is the simplest and most unifying one.[5] In the same vein, the mnemonic KISS ('Keep it simple, stupid') has become popular as an aide-memoire to the clinician to find simple explanations for medical problems.

An appreciation of the probability of a symptom being related to a diagnosis is helpful when applying Ockham's razor, as is an awareness that it is not always correct. Particularly in the ageing population, multiple independent diagnoses rather than a single unifying one may be prevalent.[5] For example, there are more common diagnoses that could be responsible for each of the symptoms that form the triad (cognitive impairment, gait disturbance and incontinence) associated with idiopathic normal pressure hydrocephalus.[6] But Ockham's razor helps us to *think* about the possibility of a unifying diagnosis and thus perhaps consider a diagnosis that might otherwise be overlooked. Sometimes a unifying explanation for multiple symptoms may be a rare disease, whereas on other occasions it may be the most common one.

Sutton's law (from the bank robber Willie Sutton) states that one should 'go for where the money is', meaning one should choose the most obvious diagnosis.[1] It can be beneficial to be aware of this principle when approaching a clinical problem since it can direct one to request investigations of the highest diagnostic value, thus saving time and money and avoiding subjecting patients to unnecessary tests.[7] However, it is important to understand its limitations. Croskerry writes that following Sutton's law can result in a failure to consider a full range of possibilities and 'a calling off of a search early when something is found,' which can lead to diagnostic error (Sutton's slip).[1]

DIAGNOSES OF EXCLUSION

Certain diagnoses can be made clinically; for example, in a reasonably well child with findings consistent with chickenpox, an initial clinical diagnosis can be made without the need for further investigation. In other cases, such as bowel symptoms suggestive of irritable bowel syndrome (IBS), we must actively rule out a number of other diagnoses such as coeliac disease and cancer before making this diagnosis. Therefore, the diagnosis of IBS is classed as a diagnosis of exclusion. The reason for this is that other more serious pathologies can mimic the symptoms and examination findings in IBS, and hence we should rule out these conditions first.

PATHOGNOMONIC FINDINGS

Pathognomonic signs and symptoms are those which are specifically indicative of a particular condition. Care needs to be exercised here, and it is best to have an appreciation of the positive predictive value of signs and symptoms rather than relying on a list of those which are deemed pathognomonic. For example, Koplik's spots (white lesions on the buccal mucosa) have long been described as pathognomonic of measles.[8] However, Koplik's spots have since been described in echovirus and parvovirus B19 illnesses.[9] Zenner and Nacul's study of measles cases in the UK found that if Koplik's spots were used as a diagnostic tool, the positive predictive value for a confirmed diagnosis of measles across hospital and primary care settings was 80%.[9] Hence Koplik's spots are a highly predictive (but not pathognomonic) finding for measles, and the authors suggest that if they are present in a case of suspected measles, the case should be treated as 'probable measles'.[9]

Therefore, a knowledge of signs and symptoms described as 'pathognomonic' for certain conditions can be helpful in terms of using them to add weight to the evidence that points towards a particular diagnosis, but they should never solely be relied on to make a diagnosis.

FORMATION OF A DIFFERENTIAL DIAGNOSIS: MEDICAL AND SURGICAL SIEVES

Medical and surgical sieves are diagnostic aids that can help in the generation of a wide list of differential diagnoses using type 2 thinking.[10] They are a type of cognitive forcing strategy (see the section on diagnostic error below). An example is the mnemonic 'INVITED MDC', which can be used to help think of possible diagnoses under different categories such as malignancy and infectious disease:

- Infection.
- Neoplasia.
- Vascular.
- Inflammatory/ autoimmune.
- Trauma.
- Endocrine.
- Degenerative.
- Metabolic.
- Drugs.
- Congenital.

(Reproduced with permission from Oxford Medical Education [http://www.oxfordmedicaleducation.com/medical-mnemonics/clinical-general-mnemonics/])

Chai *et al.* developed a 'compass medicine', which is a diagnostic aid that uses a surgical sieve approach to help generate a differential diagnosis list. It helps the user structure their diagnostic thinking. Chai *et al.*'s recent study attempted to determine the effect of using such an aid on the diagnostic ability of medical students and showed positive results.[10] However, this is an emerging field of research and there is much scope for further development of diagnostic aids and for research into their usefulness, especially in terms of their impact on reducing diagnostic error.

CLINICAL PREDICTION RULES

Clinical prediction rules use predictors from a patient's history, examination and investigations to help a clinician decide, for example, the following:

- Whether a patient has a certain diagnosis (e.g. the Wells score for prediction of deep vein thrombosis [DVT]).
- Is at risk of a diagnosis (e.g. the $ABCD^2$ rule for risk of stroke).
- Or perhaps qualifies for certain treatments (e.g. using the Centor criteria for streptococcal pharyngitis to decide whether to treat a patient with antibiotics).

Clinical prediction rules can be very helpful tools when used alongside other diagnostic strategies to improve the accuracy of diagnosis and aid decisions regarding further investigation and treatment. Keogh *et al.* recently created a register of clinical prediction rules used in primary care and found 434 rules in the literature.[11] Of these, just over half had been validated, and a very small percentage had been assessed in terms of their clinical impact.[11] Hence it is important when applying a clinical prediction rule in practice to understand the evidence base for it and thus have an appreciation of its reliability. The development of an international web-based register of clinical prediction rules will go a long way towards helping clinicians make decisions on which rules to use.[11]

Some clinical prediction rules are used widely in clinical practice. One example is the modified Wells score. Investigations are used alongside history and examination and not in place of them. Knowing when to request a test (and why) is a skill. The modified Wells scores for DVT and pulmonary embolism (PE) help to give an indication of the pretest probability that a patient has those conditions by assigning a score to the presence of certain risk factors and to whether there is an alternative diagnosis that is as or more likely. The patient is then categorised as either low, moderate or high probability of having a DVT or PE. A knowledge of this pretest probability is valuable since, as the pretest probability increases, a positive test result on investigation is more likely to be a true positive test result.[12] Hence in patients with a low probability of DVT/PE, we can avoid unnecessary (and, in the case of a CT pulmonary angiogram, potentially harmful) investigations.

DIAGNOSTIC ERROR

The term *diagnostic error* refers to situations in which a diagnosis is missed, delayed or incorrect.[13] Singh *et al.* emphasise that these situations often overlap within a single case.[14] Research in this area is an emerging field and very challenging in terms of how diagnostic error is defined and measured.[15] For example, as clinical presentations and the diagnostic process evolve over time, information gathered at a given time point may strongly support the clinician's conclusion of what may ultimately turn out to be a 'wrong diagnosis'.[15] Should this be classed as diagnostic error? Although there are obstacles, we are beginning to get a clearer picture of diagnostic error in clinical practice, and the next agenda is to develop strategies to try to prevent it.

HEURISTICS

Along with Amos Tversky, the Nobel Prize winner Daniel Kahneman introduced the concept of heuristics in his paper 'Judgement under uncertainty: heuristics and biases'.[16] Heuristics or mental shortcuts simplify the decision-making process, and a reliance on them can lead to systematic errors or 'biases'.[17] Examples of heuristics used in clinical problem solving might be visual pattern recognition, 'mindlines' (internalised guidelines), mental maps and rules of thumb, all of which are largely developed through clinical experience.[18]

COGNITIVE ERRORS

Errors in diagnosis are often categorised as being caused by systems, patient or doctor factors.[19] Cognitive errors come under the 'doctor' category and are related to the diagnostic process or the knowledge of the clinician.[13] The majority of errors, however, are due to mistakes in the decision-making process rather than due to a lack of knowledge.[20] In addition, attitudinal and affective factors such as overconfidence and fatigue feed into errors in the decision-making process. Another factor is the 'cognitive miser function' described by Croskerry as 'a tendency to default to a state that consumes fewer cognitive resources'.[21]

Cognitive errors can occur in either system 1 or system 2 thinking. It is believed that we spend the majority of time using system 1, and that most errors occur in this system as it is unconscious and less deliberate than system 2 thinking.[20] However, error can occur in system 2, from, for example, problems with hypothesis generation. Decision makers using system 1 often use heuristics or mental shortcuts that aid the decision-making process.[22] Heuristics help to bring structure to an undifferentiated problem, but when they result in faulty decisions they are described as 'cognitive bias'. Thirty types of cognitive bias identified in clinical practice have recently been catalogued.[1] In the following section we highlight selected cognitive biases.

PREMATURE CLOSURE AND ANCHORING

When a clinician thinks of an initial diagnosis, fails to fully consider alternatives and the initial diagnosis turns out to be incorrect, the process can be described as *premature closure*.[23] The clinician makes a diagnosis early on before they have gathered sufficient information to obtain the full picture.

Anchoring occurs when the clinician gives too much weight to information gained initially; for example, they may hear about a patient's cough, feel this must be due to infection and pursue that line of thought when in fact, on careful questioning, the patient would reveal some months of unintentional weight loss and a 50 pack–year smoking history. Anchoring also occurs when a diagnostic label has been applied to a patient by another clinician; this is then assumed to be correct and it becomes difficult to look at the situation from a different perspective.[24]

Kumar *et al.* recently illustrated how an aortic dissection was successfully diagnosed by avoiding premature closure (closing on a diagnosis of ischaemic heart disease) in a patient presenting with chest pain, and emphasised the importance of clinicians' scrutiny of their cognitive processes, vigilance to alternative diagnoses and the value of a comprehensive history of the presenting complaint.[23]

AVAILABILITY BIAS

This refers to the availability or ease of recall of diagnoses to form a differential diagnosis. Hence when a condition is rare or presents atypically, the clinician fails to think of the diagnosis when drawing up the differential diagnoses, so the correct diagnosis is not made or is delayed.[13] It can also occur because of the clinician's recent experience – such as having seen a case of PE the previous day – which means this diagnosis is more readily brought to mind in a patient presenting with shortness of breath.[18] To consciously avoid such bias, a balance has to be struck between drawing up long lists of differential diagnoses, giving too much weight to rare conditions and the fact that more common diagnoses are much more likely.

CONFIRMATION BIAS

A clinician sometimes sees a patient, thinks of a possible diagnosis early on and unconsciously seeks to confirm that diagnosis during the rest of the consultation. In this scenario, their mind can be closed off to other possibilities, and key features are overlooked because they do not fit with the initial diagnosis as formulated. Other information gained can be interpreted in a modified manner, again to fit with the initial diagnosis, all leading to confirmation bias.[13]

GAMBLER'S FALLACY

Each individual patient case is independent of the next (with exceptions such as the outbreak of infectious disease or mass exposure to a toxin, for example). Therefore, if a clinician has seen two cases of appendicitis that morning, the next patient presenting with abdominal pain may indeed have appendicitis too. Gambler's fallacy is a cognitive error that occurs when the clinician thinks 'I've seen two cases of appendicitis this morning, this third patient with abdominal pain MUST have something else.'[18] Each case should be given the same care and attention, and be taken on its own merits.

BASE RATE NEGLECT

This error occurs because the diagnostician fails to consider how common commonly occurring diagnoses are likely to be (the base rate). If more esoteric and less commonly occurring diagnoses are selected without evidence to support them, diagnostic error can occur.[25]

METACOGNITION AND COGNITIVE STRATEGIES TO AVOID ERROR

Brush *et al*. write that there is 'no substitute for knowledge and experience in improving diagnostic accuracy'.[22] It is stated that error occurs in up to 15% of clinical decisions; techniques to reduce error in medicine are therefore an important emerging field of research.[26] Complementing a sound background knowledge and clinical experience, the development and practising of skills of metacognition (i.e. thinking critically about our thinking and then reflecting on the processes in our decision making) may make a contribution to improving diagnostic accuracy. Cognitive strategies appropriately applied to decision-making processes and taught in medical education may also help to reduce error.

Croskerry describes an 'executive override' function between system 1 and 2 thinking that can allow system 2 to make checks on the decision being made and, as part of this, could include cognitive debiasing (i.e. checking whether our thinking has been biased by the commonly encountered cognitive biases in medical diagnosis and implementing a change to avoid such bias). For example, this might cause us to check whether we have considered all possibilities in the differential diagnosis or whether we have been subject to premature closure. Broadly, cognitive strategies can be divided into educational strategies (to help the clinician become more aware of the decision-making process and pitfalls within it) and workplace strategies (to be used during the diagnostic process itself).[27] Workplace strategies include checklists (general, symptom-specific, debiasing and those to aid differential diagnoses), cognitive forcing strategies (that ask the clinician to look again or reconsider their diagnoses, for example) and guided reflection (to promote more reflection 'in the moment' rather than in hindsight).[27]

Dual process cognitive interventions to enhance diagnostic reasoning have recently been systematically reviewed.[27] This has provided some evidence for the efficacy of specific cognitive forcing strategies and for guided reflection, but we have no evidence yet for real workplace effects of these interventions.[27] This field of research is young and methodologically challenging but could have great impact on the training of future clinicians and thus patient care in the future.

SUMMARY

- This chapter explores the factors that affect clinical decision making and explains that selected strategies will be discussed more fully in individual chapters.
- These selected strategies are spot diagnosis (used in the initiation phase), pattern recognition trigger and pattern recognition fit (used in the initiation and refinement stages), red and yellow flags (used in the initiation and refinement stages), restricted rule-outs (used in the refinement phase), probabilistic reasoning (used in the refinement stage), test of time (used in the final diagnosis stage) and test of treatment (used in the final diagnosis stage).
- Additional strategies and diagnostic aids are explained, such as Ockham's (Occam's) razor, Sutton's law, diagnoses of exclusion, pathognomonic findings, medical and surgical sieves, and clinical prediction rules.
- The final section discusses in more depth the subject of diagnostic error, heuristics and cognitive bias. Selected cognitive errors (premature closure, anchoring, availability bias, confirmation bias, gambler's fallacy, base rate neglect and cognitive miser function) are highlighted, concluding with a brief discussion on whether metacognition and cognitive strategies can be used to avoid diagnostic error.

REFERENCES

1 Croskerry P. Achieving quality in clinical decision making: cognitive strategies and detection of bias. *Acad Emerg Med* 2002;**9**:1184–204.

2 Heneghan C, Glasziou P, Thompson M, *et al.* Diagnostic strategies used in primary care. *BMJ* 2009;**338**:b946.

3 Adams E, Goyder C, Heneghan C, Brand L, Aijawi R. Clinical reasoning of junior doctors in emergency medicine: a grounded theory study. *Emerg Med J* 2017;**34:**70–5.

4 Balla J, Heneghan C, Thompson M, Balla M. Clinical decision making in a high-risk primary care environment: a qualitative study in the UK. *BMJ Open* 2012;**2**:e000414.

5 Wardrop D. Ockham's Razor: sharpen or re-sheathe? *J Roy Soc Med* 2008;**101**:50–1.

6 Lakhan SE, Gross K. The triad of idiopathic normal-pressure hydrocephalus: a clinical practice case report. *Libyan J Med* 2008;**3**:54–7.

7 Watanuki S, Honda H, Minemura N, *et al.* Sutton's law: keep going where the money is. *J Gen Intern Med* 2015;**30**:1711–15.

8 Cockbain BC, Bharucha T, Irish D, Jacobs M. Measles in older children and adults. *BMJ* 2017;**356**:j426.

9 Zenner D, Nacul L. Predictive power of Koplik's spots for the diagnosis of measles. *J Infect Dev Ctries* 2011;**6**:271–5.

10 Chai J, Evans L, Hughes T. Diagnostc aids: the surgical sieve revisited. *Clin Teach* 2017;**14**:263–7.

11 Keogh C, Wallace E, O'Brien KK, *et al.* Developing an international register of clinical prediction rules for use in primary care: a descriptive analysis. *Ann Fam Med* 2014;**12**:359–66.

12 Kelly J, Hunt BJ. The utility of pretest probability assessment in patients with clinically suspected venous thromboembolism. *J Thromb Haemost* 2003;**1**:1888–96.

13 Phua DH, Tan NC. Cognitive aspects of diagnostic errors. *Ann Acad Med Singapore* 2013;**42**:33–41.

14   Singh H, Schiff GD, Graber ML, Onakpoya I, Thompson MJ. The global burden of diagnostic errors in primary care. *BMJ Qual Saf* 2017;**26**:484.

15   Zwaan L, Singh H. The challenges in defining and measuring diagnostic error. *Diagnosis (Berl)* 2015;**2**:97–103.

16   Tversky A, Kahneman D. Judgment under uncertainty: heuristics and biases. *Science* 1974;**185**:1124.

17   Kahneman D. *Thinking, Fast and Slow*. London: Penguin; 2011.

18   Bate L, Hutchinson A, Underhill J, Maskrey N. How clinical decisions are made. *Br J Clin Pharmacol* 2012;**74**:614–20.

19   Goyder CR, Jones CHD, Heneghan CJ, Thompson MJ. Missed opportunities for diagnosis: lessons learned from diagnostic errors in primary care. *Br J Gen Pract* 2015;**65**:e838–e844.

20   Croskerry P, Singhal G, Mamede S. Cognitive debiasing 1: origins of bias and theory of debiasing. *BMJ Qual Saf* 2013;**22**:ii58–ii64.

21   Croskerry P. Clinical cognition and diagnostic error: applications of a dual process model of reasoning. *Adv Health Sci Educ* 2009;**14**(Suppl 1):27–35.

22   Brush JE, Jr., Sherbino J, Norman GR. How expert clinicians intuitively recognize a medical diagnosis. *Am J Med* 2017;**130**:629–34.

23   Kumar B, Kanna B, Kumar S. The pitfalls of premature closure: clinical decision-making in a case of aortic dissection. *BMJ Case Rep* 2011;**2011**:bcr0820114594.

24   Bhatti A. Cognitive bias in clinical practice – nurturing healthy skepticism among medical students. *Adv Med Educ Pract* 2018;**9**:235–7.

25   Pinnock R, Welch P. Learning clinical reasoning. *J Paediatr Child Health* 2014;**50**:253–7.

26   Croskerry P. When I say … cognitive debiasing. *Med Educ* 2015;**49**:656–7.

27   Lambe KA, Reilly G, Kelly BD, Curristan S. Dual-process cognitive interventions to enhance diagnostic reasoning: a systematic review. *BMJ Qual Saf* 2016;**25**:808.

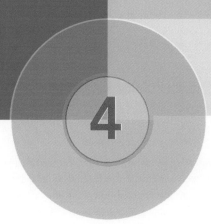

The history

4

INTRODUCTION

The history is an integral part of clinical diagnosis and arguably the most fundamental, determining the subsequent examination and appropriate investigations.[1] The history usually comes from the patient but if this is not possible (e.g. if the patient is unable to communicate or is a young child), other sources such as next of kin, carers, witnesses and allied health professionals may provide a valuable history. The key features of a good history are governed by the clinical context but in general are:

- Patient-centred, helping to establish rapport and build a relationship with the patient.
- Accurate.
- Comprehensive.
- Relevant to the clinical condition and context.
- Taken in a timely manner and consolidated by the clinician such that the salient points can be relayed to colleagues.

INFORMATION GATHERING

Whenever possible, take the history from a patient yourself rather than relying on others – this may help avoid cognitive biases such as premature closure and anchoring (see Chapter 3).[2] Eliciting a structured history is key.

At medical school, the structured approach of presenting complaint, history of presenting complaint, past medical history, drug history, allergies, social history, family history and systems enquiry is usually taught. After qualification, the approach becomes increasingly tailored to the clinical context, knowledge and experience of the clinician. For example, in UK primary care, where details of a patient's past medical history and medication are likely to be available, the approach will be very different from that of emergency department clerking, where there may be no prior information. Similarly, the approach will be adapted in the context of telephone triage, where the consultation lacks the benefit of being able to pick up on important non-verbal cues.

Under the umbrella of 'social history' are a number of important lines of enquiry such as home situation, intimate relationships, alcohol and smoking history, occupation and travel history. It is extremely useful here to try to ascertain the impact of the patient's symptoms on their activities of daily living and what, if any, support they have.[1]

It is important whenever possible that the patient is able to describe their symptoms and give their narrative in their own words. Patients really appreciate time to explain and feeling they are listened to. Active and attentive listening is a key skill, and sitting face to face with the patient can be very helpful in this respect.[3] Wieling describes the process as 'history building with the patient' rather than 'taking a history from a patient'.[3]

There is a skill in not becoming distracted by seemingly irrelevant aspects of the history, although the wise clinician will be cautious in prematurely discarding any aspect of the patient's account. The development of a good rapport with a patient helps to engender trust and facilitate the gathering of accurate information.[4] Follow-up questions aid the exploration of the presenting complaint, and the clinician can then explore further what the patient means by the symptoms they describe (e.g. what does the patient actually mean by 'feeling faint'?). If a patient's answers seem unclear, consider whether questions need to be reframed or whether you are pushing too hard for a clear description of symptoms that cannot be described in more detail.

SPECIFIC APPROACHES IN HISTORY TAKING

We do not attempt to provide a comprehensive guide to history taking in this chapter or explore the vast area of communication skills that are intergral to the process of history taking; instead, we consider specific approaches that can be employed when gathering information from patients.

SELF-LABELLING

When taking a history, it can be very useful to glean from the patient what they think is causing their symptoms. 'Self-labelling' (or self-diagnosis) is the term used to describe this strategy, in which a patient offers what they think the diagnosis may be.[5] This may occur at the start of a consultation or clerking, for example 'I am having a flare-up of my asthma', or it may be elicited when the patient is asked about their ideas, concerns and expectations, for example 'My father had a spot on the end of his nose and it turned out to be a skin cancer.' Situations in which self-labelling causes harm occur when patients wrongly self-diagnose and perhaps do not present early with the problem.[6]

Recurrent diagnoses (e.g. recurrent urinary tract infection) tend to be self-diagnosed most accurately, although there is little research in this area.[6] Self-labelling is useful not only in informing the clinician's approach to history taking, but also in helping to address the patient's concerns. It is essential to consider a patient's 'self-diagnosis' objectively. Is it correct? Is their suggestion possible or is it for whatever reason unlikely in your opinion? With the benefit of the Internet, self-labelling is more prevalent and hence it is useful to explore why and how the patient has come to their conclusions.

Occasionally, when asked their view on what might be causing their symptoms, a patient will reply with words to the effect of 'You're the doctor – you tell me.' Do not be dismayed by this or any other apparently prickly response. It provides a useful insight into the patient's approach to the consultation and suggests that you may have to work to achieve shared decision making.

THINKING AND LISTENING USING 'LINKED QUESTIONS'

Thrush makes the point that history taking should be detective work rather than a mechanical task.[1] While listening to the patient, the clinician is also thinking about what the next questions should be and how they can be used to refine a differential diagnosis. The more experienced clinician generates hypotheses and tests them with specific questions while taking the history. The presenting symptoms should trigger sets of questions to help assess the likelihood that, for example, a myocardial infarction has caused chest pain. In a patient presenting with chest pain that might be cardiac in origin, after taking a full history of the pain, the following questions should be asked:

- 'Do you have high blood pressure?'
- 'Do you have diabetes?'
- 'Do you smoke?'/'Have you ever smoked?'
- 'Do you have high cholesterol? Have you had it tested?'
- 'Have you ever had angina or heart problems in the past?'
- 'Has anyone in your family had a heart attack at a young age? Below the age of 60?'
- 'What is your work?'
- 'Do you get much in the way of exercise?'

Questions for vascular problems include:

- 'Have you ever had a stroke or mini stroke (TIA – transient ischaemic attack)?'
- 'Do you ever get any pain in your calves when walking?'

MNEMONICS

'Set piece questions' (often remembered by a mnemonic) to expand and further explore a presenting complaint can be helpful to ensure comprehensive information gathering. SOCRATES is a classic example of a mnemonic used to explore pain. For the patient who says, 'I have tummy pain', the items will be:

- Site: 'Where is the pain?'
- Onset: 'Does the pain come on suddenly or gradually?'
- Character: 'Can you describe what it feels like?'
- Radiation: 'Does the pain go anywhere else?'
- Associated symptoms: 'Is there anything else you notice at the same time?'
- Timing: 'How long did the pain last, and does it occur at any particular time?'
- Exacerbating and relieving factors: 'Is there anything that seems to make the pain better or worse?'
- Severity: 'On a scale of 0 to 10, with 10 being the worst pain, how would you rate the pain?' Or if you prefer not to ask for a numerical value 'How does this pain compare in severity with other pain you have experienced?'

The use of mnemonics can be seen as a debiasing strategy as they are a cognitive aid that can help to increase the accuracy of clinical decisions.[7] However, remember that mnemonics do not cover all possibilities and, if reeled off as a list of questions, can interfere with the flow of the conversation and the development of rapport with the patient. The skilled clinician will ask a patient to tell their story in full, then summarise the patient's symptoms back to them for confirmation before going on to ask specific additional questions to develop a comprehensive history.

A 63-year-old woman presents with the following: 'I've been having problems with numbness in my hand. It's always the left hand and I am constantly shaking it to make it feel better. I thought I might have slept on it but it keeps happening. I am noticing it at work now so I thought I should come and get it checked out.'

The first step is to fully explore the presenting complaint. Remember to listen to as much of the patient's opening comments as possible without interruption. Then ask some questions to clarify. Find out exactly what the patient means by 'numbness' by asking 'Can you tell me more about what the numbness feels like?' or 'What do you mean by "numbness"?'

The patient volunteers that it feels 'like a tingling, like pins and needles'. The description is of paraesthesia, and the lesion could be anywhere from the sensory cortex to the peripheral sensory nerve.[8] With all potentially neurological symptoms, it is helpful to explore the presentation in such a way that the lesion can first be localised in general terms (i.e. whether this is a problem with the central nervous system or peripheral nervous system and, if peripheral, whether it is a nerve or muscle problem).[1] In addition, the onset, duration and progression of the symptoms are important to ascertain whether this is an acute, subacute or chronic problem.[1]

1 What further clarification questions would you ask about the presenting complaint?

Perhaps clarify 'Are your symptoms only occurring in your left hand?', since distinguishing between unilateral and bilateral paraesthesia significantly helps in formulating a differential diagnosis. For example, if there is bilateral paraesthesia in the hands with no motor involvement, we should be thinking about the causes of a peripheral sensory neuropathy. It is also useful to ask what the patient is doing when their symptoms come on.

In addition, asking 'Which part of the hand do you get the symptoms in?', 'Are the symptoms localised to the hand or do they spread up the arm?' and 'Do you get symptoms elsewhere in the body?' will help to further localise any lesion.

The patient volunteers that the symptoms are localised and occur only in her left hand. This helps to narrow the differential diagnosis further.

The patient is presenting with a sensory symptom. It is important to ask about motor deficit. A general question such as 'Have you noticed any other problems with your hand?' can be helpful in order to avoid directly leading a patient regarding weakness.

The patient reports that she plays the piano at home and has recently found playing with her left hand more difficult.

An exploration of symptoms should include exacerbating and relieving factors. Given what the patient has told us, the history points to a mixed sensory and motor problem, localised to the left hand.

The information above points towards a problem with a peripheral nerve. It is important to use the history and examination to localise the lesion further to a specific nerve.

Carpal tunnel syndrome (CTS) would fit with the symptoms and is high on the differential diagnosis list.

2 Apart from your main diagnosis, what else might be on the differential diagnosis list?

Ulnar neuropathy is a differential diagnosis. This may be caused by compression where the ulnar nerve crosses the medial humeral epicondyle, which would cause similar symptoms (cubital tunnel syndrome), or runs through Guyon's canal.[8,9] However, with an ulnar neuropathy, the paraesthesia is felt in the little finger and the medial half of the ring finger, and the motor deficit corresponds to muscles supplied by the ulnar nerve (you can therefore, for example, test finger abduction against resistance, which tests the interosseus muscles).

Pronator teres syndrome is possible also but it is much rarer.[10] This is compression of the median nerve between the two heads of the pronator teres. The clinical picture is of pain, numbness or paraesthesia in the anterior forearm as well as the hand, whereas these symptoms are localised to the hand (the palmar lateral three and a half digits) in CTS.[11]

CTS is high on the list of differential diagnoses, but try to avoid confirmation bias or the misdiagnosis of another nerve entrapment syndrome or polyneuropathy as CTS. Avoid this by a full sensory examination of the hand and testing aspects of motor function that help you discriminate between the ulnar, median and radial nerves. Testing thumb abduction tests abductor pollicis brevis, which is supplied by the median nerve. Testing wrist extension tests the carpi ulnaris, which is supplied by the radial nerve. As described above, assessing finger abduction tests the ulnar nerve. Testing all three nerves in the above case helps you to be more confident that you have localised the lesion to a specific nerve.

The radial nerve can be damaged secondary to humeral fracture or trauma and can be compressed at the spiral groove of the humerus.[12] A radial nerve palsy would present with wrist drop, difficulty of extension of the metacarpophalangeal joints and lack of sensation in the lateral three and a half digits and over the dorsum of the hand.[12]

To complete your assessment, check also that there are no lower limb sensory symptoms and signs.

As discussed above, remember to assess the impact of the symptoms on the patient's life. 'Are you right or left handed?' is a question that is particularly helpful for neurological problems. Also ask about occupation and activities of daily living. There are some classic symptoms that a patient may describe in relation to CTS that can help point towards the diagnosis. For example, when asked, 'Are your symptoms worse at any particular time of day?,' they may reply, 'Yes. It wakes me up at night. My hand is painful and very tingly. It is disturbing my sleep. I wake up and find I need to shake my hand and arm to make it feel better.'

This is a description of the 'flick sign', which has been found to be highly sensitive and specific (>90%) for CTS.[13] However, remember that patients do not necessarily have to present with the classic symptoms and features of a certain condition. Beware the atypical presentation. In fact, it is reported that atypical presentations of aortic dissection are more common than the classic description.[14]

In the above case, past medical history and social history can add some important information and may point to possible causes for CTS. It is important to identify a cause as it may be treatable (e.g. diabetes mellitus).

3 What conditions may predispose to the development of the most likely diagnosis here?

- Trauma to the nerve, for example caused by operation of vibrating machinery or hand tools.[8]
- Sleeping with the wrist hyperflexed (which compromises the vascular supply to the nerve).[8]
- Obesity.
- Diabetes mellitus.
- Hypothyroidism.
- Acromegaly.
- Pregnancy.
- Rheumatoid arthritis.

Sometimes patients point towards a correct diagnosis by 'self-labelling' (as discussed above), and this can be explored as part of determining the patient's 'ideas, concerns and expectations'.

For example, on asking 'Do you have any thoughts as to what might be causing this?,' the patient replies: 'My mum has had an operation for carpal tunnel and she said it really sounds like the same thing.' Sometimes, however, their concerns will be misplaced; for example, 'My grandmother has been having mini strokes and I was worried this might be a similar thing.'

Next, with the differential diagnosis of a localised neuropathy in mind, you examine the patient's hands.

4 Would you expect to find anything on inspection of the hands?

Remember to compare the patient's right and left hands. If the condition has been long-standing and untreated, you may find wasting of the thenar eminence (**Figure 4.1**). You should also inspect for any precipitating factors such as injury, oedema or signs of arthritis.[13]

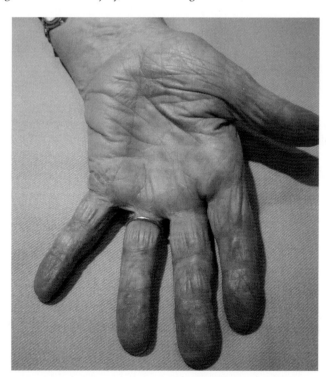

Fig. 4.1 Wasting of the thenar eminence of the left hand of a female patient with chronic CTS.

5 What might be found on neurological examination of the upper limbs?

A sensory deficit in the median nerve distribution and signs of motor deficit in the 'LOAF' muscles (lateral two lumbricals, opponens pollicis, abductor pollicis brevis and flexor pollicis brevis), which are innervated by the median nerve, may be found. Note the discussion above regarding fully assessing the radial and ulnar nerves in the hand as part of your examination.

6 What tests can be performed during the examination?

Phalen's, Tinel's and the hand elevation tests are provocation tests since they are manoeuvres that can reproduce the patient's symptoms. When performing them, be careful not to cause pain. Phalen's and Tinel's tests work by causing compression (venous engorgement in the case of Phalen's test) of the median nerve in the carpal tunnel. In the hand elevation test, the patient raises their arm above their hand for 1 minute. These tests have similar sensitivity and specificity (Phalen's test, sensitivity 57–68%, specificity 58–73%; Tinel's text, sensitivity 36–50%, specificity 77%).[13] However, there is a debate in the literature, and other published research suggests these tests have little or no diagnostic value.[15] The 'flick sign' is yet to be validated.

On examination of the patient described here, there are no signs of weakness but Phalen's test is positive. The history is most consistent with CTS.

7 How might the diagnosis be confirmed?

Here we could use a 'test of treatment' strategy (see Chapter 10) to help confirm the diagnosis. Nocturnal immobilisation with a splint is first-line treatment, and there is also evidence that corticosteroid injection into the carpal tunnel provides effective short-term relief.[16]

Nerve conduction studies are sometimes used to help aid diagnosis when splints and corticosteroid injections are ineffective.

8 What further treatment options are available?

Surgical decompression, which involves dividing the flexor retinaculum (a carpal tunnel release procedure), can be used in patients who do not respond to conservative management. When examining a patient's hands, look for these scars (**Figures 4.2** and **4.3**) – they are very relevant in finals and other professional OSCE-based exams.

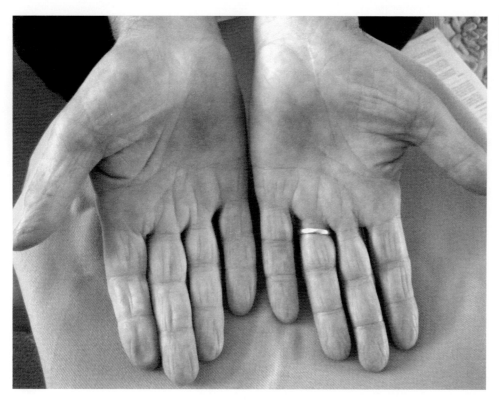

Fig. 4.2 Carpal tunnel release procedure scar at the left wrist.

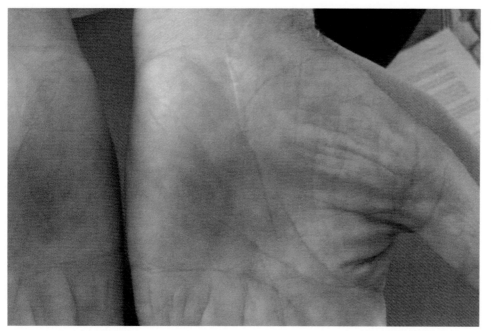

Fig. 4.3 Close-up of the scar.

A 30-year-old woman presents to her GP with a history of malaise and fatigue. The patient is new to the surgery.

She reports that this has been going on for the last 3–4 months and in particular she feels a lack of energy at work (she is a PE teacher). She also complains that she is tired in the evenings and has a decreased appetite. She has felt intermittently nauseated and thinks she has probably lost weight. When asked about her concerns, she reports that she 'is unsure what is causing her tiredness but just wants to feel normal again'.

Non-specific symptoms in the presenting complaint are a challenge. The symptom 'fatigue' has a wide differential diagnosis and it can be difficult to approach it in a systematic manner. It is a symptom to which in up to 43% of cases no diagnostic label can be attached.[17] One approach is to think of patients with fatigue as falling into the categories shown in **Figure 4.4**.

Fig. 4.4 Thinking about the causes of 'fatigue' (adapted from ideas from Wilson *et al.* and Jones *et al.*[17,18]).

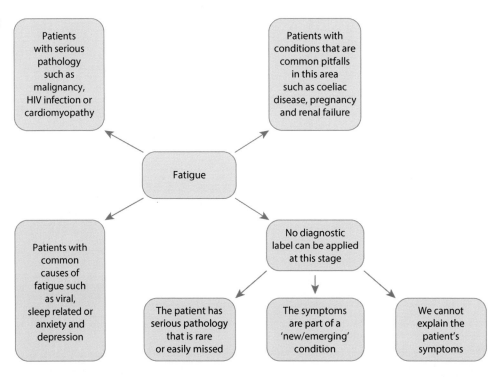

Jones *et al.* describe a diagnostic label as a label referring to a working diagnosis on which further investigation or treatment might be based, or a label that is a marker of symptoms that do not have serious underlying pathology (once they have been ruled out).[18]

1 Are there any red flags in this patient's history?

In the above history, the patient complains of unintentional weight loss. This may be a symptom of serious pathology such as malignancy, hyperthyroidism or diabetes mellitus.

2 What other features in a history might be a red flag in patients presenting with fatigue?

Wilson *et al.* suggest that the following are potential red flags in individuals presenting with fatigue:

- Unintentional weight loss.
- Abnormal bleeding.
- Shortness of breath.
- Fever.
- Tiredness that is of recent onset in an older person.

3 What questions might help to determine if this patient's symptoms are due to some of the more common causes of tiredness?

Here, think about anxiety and depression, lifestyle factors such as sleep, alcohol and work, and viral infections as causes of fatigue:

- 'How is your mood?'
- 'How are things at home?'
- 'How are these symptoms affecting you?'
- 'Have you ever had any problems with anxiety and/or depression in the past?'
- 'Have you recently been unwell?'
- 'Have you had a sore throat, runny nose or cough?'
- 'How is your sleep?', 'How much do you sleep?'
- 'Do you drink alcohol?', 'How much alcohol do you drink in a typical week?'
- 'Do you smoke?', 'Do you ever use any recreational drugs?'

We know this patient is a PE teacher. It is important to ask about occupation as work-related stress and shift work can have a big impact on a patient's feeling of well-being and on symptoms of fatigue.

The patient felt that her sleep was 'OK'. She reported that she had been going to bed earlier but it had not made much difference. She is not currently in a relationship and she reports that she could not be pregnant. She tries to lead a healthy lifestyle, drinks very little alcohol and is a non-smoker. She tells you that although she is getting fed up with her symptoms, her mood has not been significantly affected.

She reports no positive family history for any conditions. Her parents are in their 60s and are in good health.

4 How might your examination be focused to help determine a cause for her fatigue?

Think about the elements of the physical examination and how they might be related to pathologies that can cause fatigue (*Table 4.1*).

Table 4.1 Features in the examination related to fatigue

Feature to be examined	Relationship to pathology causing fatigue
Heart rate	Tachycardia may indicate hyperthyroidism or anaemia. Bradycardia may indicate hypothyroidism
Blood pressure	Hypertension or hypotension may be related to endocrine pathologies
Pallor	Pale conjunctivae and nails related to anaemia
Temperature	Fever indicating infection
Weight	Measure weight to help assess for cachexia, hyperthyroidism, hypothyroidism, coeliac disease, etc. It will be useful to have a baseline for comparative purposes at follow-up
Thyroid	Look for signs of a goitre or thyroid swelling (hyperthyroidism and malignancy as causes of weight loss, hypothyroidism as a cause of weight gain). Also look for a tremor and lid lag
Lymphadenopathy	The presence of lymphadenopathy may indicate the presence of infection or malignancy
Cardiovascular and respiratory examination	Think about how problems in the cardiovascular and respiratory systems might cause fatigue. Are there signs of heart failure? Are there signs of lung pathologies, for example chronic pulmonary emboli or pulmonary fibrosis?
Abdomen	Check for hepatosplenomegaly associated with liver disorders and malignancy

5 You examine the patient and start with her hands. What observations do you make from Figure 4.5?

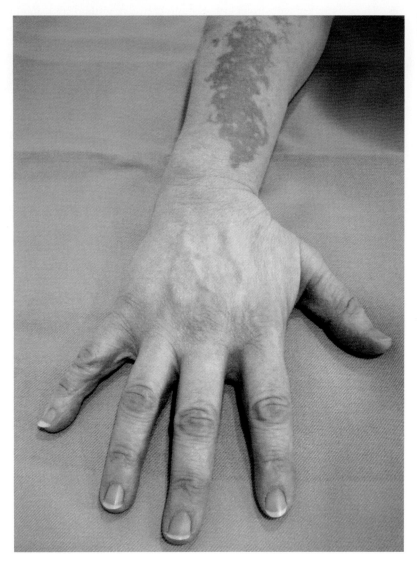

Fig. 4.5 The patient's right hand.

This right hand in **Figure 4.5** is that of a young woman. The skin and nails are in good condition. The patient has some discoloration of the forearm. Is the cause of this discoloration hyperpigmentation of the skin, hypopigmentation (paler skin) on the rest of the arm, depigmentation (absence of melanin) on the rest of the arm or pigmentation of some other kind (e.g. haemosiderin deposition)?[19]

On examination, the patient looks reasonably thin but in good health. Observations are normal and you do not find any signs apart from the skin signs above. You ask the patient to tell you more about her skin. She tells you that she was diagnosed with vitiligo 2 years ago. Her condition is more noticeable during the summer.

6 Could the presence of vitiligo be a potential clue to the cause of this patient's fatigue?

Yes. There is a known strong association between vitiligo and autoimmune thyroid disease.[20] Vitiligo is found as part of the rare autoimmune polyendocrine syndromes and is also associated with systemic lupus erythematosus, rheumatoid arthritis, inflammatory bowel disease, pernicious anaemia and Addison's disease.[20,21]

You have not found anything else untoward on examination, and the history does not point to a specific cause at this stage.

7 What investigations would you request in the first instance and why?

It would be sensible to request a urine dipstick test to look for glycosuria, and hence diabetes mellitus, as a cause of fatigue and weight loss. You might also request a full blood count (FBC), urea and electrolytes, liver function, calcium, thyroid function and anti-tissue transglutaminase (anti-TTG) antibodies to look for signs of infection, anaemia, haematological malignancy, renal dysfunction, liver dysfunction, hypercalcaemia, thyroid disease and coeliac disease as causes of fatigue and nausea.

8 What measures could you suggest to the patient in the first instance to help her with her symptoms and aid the diagnostic process?

At this stage, it would be useful to ask the patient to keep a diary of her symptoms so that any emerging patterns may be discerned. In addition, you could give her a patient information leaflet relating to sleep hygiene and ask her to follow the advice there as a 'test of treatment' strategy (see Chapter 10) to help determine if sleep is a major issue. You should review the patient and her results.

A week later, the patient returns to discuss the results of the investigations:

- Urinalysis is negative.
- FBC reveals haemoglobin 110 g/L, mean cell volume 78 fL.
- Na^+ 130 mmol/L, K^+ 3.5 mmol/L.
- All other blood results are normal, including anti-TTG, which is negative.

The patient reports that she had tried hard to follow good sleep hygiene but has still had bouts of feeling nauseated, and overall her symptoms are unchanged.

At this point, the patient is falling into the category of 'patient with persistent symptoms, still requiring investigation' (see **Figure 4.4**, page 28). Jones *et al.* have subcategorised this group of patients into the following:

1 The patient has a condition which at this stage has not been revealed (perhaps because it is a rare condition or because its presentation is insidious).
2 The patient has symptoms that at present we are unable to explain.[18]
3 The patient has a new or emerging condition that the medical profession is just learning about.

9 Is there a rare disease that might account for the patient's symptoms and might be associated with vitiligo? What investigation might you request?

The patient's GP suspected Addison's disease. In primary care, a 9:00 a.m. cortisol was requested, which was below the normal range. The patient was referred to an endocrinologist and the diagnosis was confirmed with a positive autoantibody titre and an elevated adrenocorticotropic hormone (ACTH) concentration.

10 How else might your suspected condition present?

This condition can present acutely with an adrenal crisis. This is characterised by hypotension and shock, hyponatraemia with hyperkalaemia and symptoms such as nausea, vomiting and abdominal pain.

PRIMARY ADRENAL INSUFFICIENCY

Primary adrenal insufficiency is also known as Addison's disease. This can be a difficult condition to diagnose since it is rare (affecting 1 in 10,000 in the UK) and is often insidious, leading to delayed diagnosis.[21] At diagnosis, 8.5% of patients with autoimmune Addison's disease have vitiligo.[21] Around 90% of patients have a marginally reduced sodium level at diagnosis, but only approximately 50% of patients have hyperkalaemia at diagnosis.[22] A recent consensus statement recommends that Addison's disease is considered in patients presenting with unexplained vomiting, diarrhoea, collapse or hypotension.[22] On examination, hyperpigmentation, particularly in the palmar creases and buccal mucosa (a result of elevated ACTH levels), should raise suspicion. The diagnosis should also be considered if laboratory investigations show the classic combination of hyponatraemia and hyperkalaemia, or there is acidosis and/or hypoglycaemia.[22]

11 Another patient who has a diagnosis of Addison's disease is shown (Figure 4.6). What features do you notice?

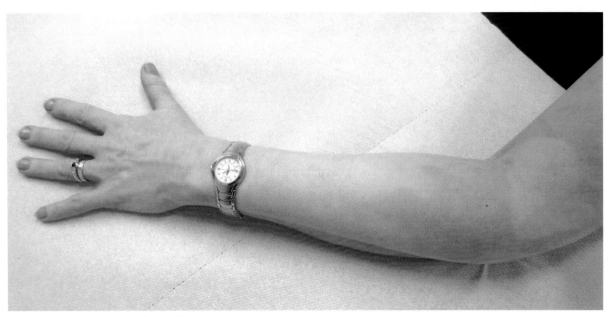

Fig. 4.6 The patient with Addison's disease.

This is a female patient. She is wearing a wedding ring on the ring finger. Her skin and nails are in good condition but there is evidence of vitiligo on the upper forearm. She is wearing a medical alert watch (**Figure 4.7**).

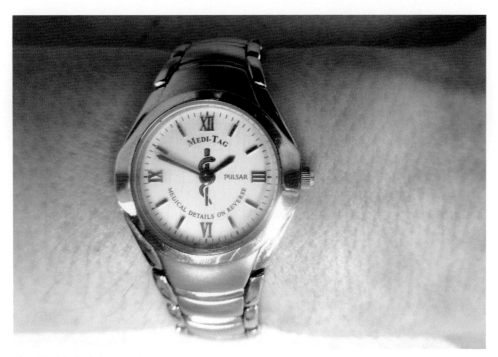

Fig. 4.7 Medical alert watch.

12 What is the reason for the medical alert watch?

Patients with Addison's disease are treated lifelong with hydrocortisone (corticosteroid) and fludrocortisone (mineralocorticoid). As their body cannot produce its own steroids, they need to match the increased steroid requirements of the body during times of stress by increasing their dose. This leads to 'sick day rules'. If a patient fails to provide their body with enough steroid (perhaps due to underdosing in times of intercurrent illness or poor compliance), an adrenal crisis can occur. In an emergency situation such as this, the medical alert watch serves to make health professionals aware of the patient's needs, ensuring prompt and appropriate treatment.

SUMMARY

- This chapter explains the key features of a good history: patient-centred, establishing rapport, building a good relationship with the patient, accurate, comprehensive and relevant to the clinical condition and context.
- It discusses the art of information gathering and describes specific approaches to history taking, such as self-labelling, linked questions and mnemonics.
- Two cases consolidate these ideas. The first is a case of carpal tunnel syndrome, and the second a patient with fatigue and vitiligo who is found to have Addison's disease.

REFERENCES

1 Thrush D. Take a good history. *Pract Neurol* 2002;**2**:113.
2 Bhatti A. Cognitive bias in clinical practice – nurturing healthy skepticism among medical students. *Adv Med Educ Pract* 2018;**9**:235–7.
3 Wieling W, van Dijk N, de Lange FJ, *et al*. History taking as a diagnostic test in patients with syncope: developing expertise in syncope. *Eur Heart J* 2015;**36**:277–80.
4 Gruppen LD. Clinical reasoning: defining it, teaching it, assessing it, studying it. *West J Emerg Med* 2017;**18**:4–7.
5 Heneghan C, Glasziou P, Thompson M, *et al*. Diagnostic strategies used in primary care. *BMJ* 2009;**338**:b946.
6 Goyder C, McPherson A, Glasziou P. Diagnosis in general practice. Self diagnosis. *BMJ* 2009;**339**:b4418.
7 Croskerry P, Nimmo G. Better clinical decision making and reducing diagnostic error. *J R Coll Physicians Edinb* 2011;**41**:155–62.
8 Beran R. Paraesthesia and peripheral neuropathy. *Aust Fam Physician* 2015;**44**:92–5.
9 Dy CJ, Mackinnon SE. Ulnar neuropathy: evaluation and management. *Curr Rev Musculoskelet Med* 2016;**9**:178–84.
10 Lee HJ, Kim I, Hong JT, Kim MS. Early surgical treatment of pronator teres syndrome. *J Korean Neurosurg Soc* 2014;**55**:296–9.
11 Asheghan M, Hollisaz MT, Aghdam AS, Khatibiaghda A. The prevalence of pronator teres among patients with carpal tunnel syndrome: cross-sectional study. *Int J Biomed Sci* 2016;**12**:89–94.
12 Bumbasirevic M, Palibrk T, Lesic A, Atkinson HDE. Radial nerve palsy. *EFORT Open Rev* 2016;**1**:286–94.
13 Wipperman J. Carpal tunnel syndrome: diagnosis and management. *Am Fam Phys* 2016;**94**:993–9.
14 Kumar B, Kanna B, Kumar S. The pitfalls of premature closure: clinical decision-making in a case of aortic dissection. *BMJ Case Rep* 2011;2011:bcr.08.2011.4594.
15 D'Arcy CA, McGee S. Does this patient have carpal tunnel syndrome? *JAMA* 2000;**283**:3110–17.
16 Marshall SC, Tardif G, Ashworth NL. Local corticosteroid injection for carpal tunnel syndrome. *Cochrane Database Syst Rev* 2007;**April 18(2)**:CD001554.
17 Wilson J, Morgan S, Magin P, van Driel M. Fatigue – a rational approach to investigation. *Aust Fam Physician* 2014;**43**:457–61.

18 Jones R, Barraclough K, Dowrick C. When no diagnostic label is applied. *BMJ* 2010;**340**:c2683.

19 Yi Zhen Chiang N, Verbov J. *Dermatology: A Handbook for Medical Students and Junior Doctors*. London: British Association of Dermatologists; 2014.

20 Baldini E, Odorisio T, Sorrenti S, *et al*. Vitiligo and autoimmune thyroid disorders. *Front Endocrinol* 2017;**8**:290.

21 Burton C, Cottrell E, Edwards J. Addison's disease: identification and management in primary care. *Br J Gen Pract* 2015;**65**:488–90.

22 Husebye ES, Allolio B, Arlt W, *et al*. Consensus statement on the diagnosis, treatment and follow-up of patients with primary adrenal insufficiency. *J Intern Med* 2013;**275**:104–15.

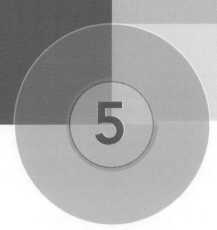

The examination

INTRODUCTION

With the development of increasingly sophisticated and specific investigations, a debate over the relevance and utility of the clinical examination has emerged.[1] Some diagnoses can be confidently made on the basis of history and examination. In other circumstances, physical examination can be viewed as a key step in refining the differential diagnosis list in order that a more judicious decision can be made with regard to which (if any) further investigations are required.[2-4] Additionally, the presence or absence of certain physical signs can help determine a patient's prognosis.[4] A careful and appropriate physical examination can therefore aid the diagnostic process and prevent unnecessary cost and burden on patients and healthcare systems.

Achieving and maintaining proficiency in physical examination is an ongoing process requiring the practising of clinical skills from medical school through to postgraduate training and beyond.[3] The honing of physical examination skills requires repetition of examination in the clinical environment, as well as study (so one knows what to look for), and can also involve simulation. It should also include feedback from peers, educators and patients.

This book is not aiming to teach 'how to examine' but we emphasise the importance of keen observation alongside a methodical and focused approach. A focused examination means one which is appropriate to the individual patient in any given clinical context and seeks answers to specific questions (such as 'Does this patient have respiratory signs that tie in with their history of shortness of breath?'). Garibaldi and Olson refer to this tailored examination as 'the hypothesis-driven examination'.[4] It incorporates the above, coupled with an appreciation of the discriminatory or diagnostic value of the manoeuvres performed.[4]

EVIDENCE-BASED EXAMINATION

An evidence-based approach to examination requires a knowledge of how the probability of a diagnosis is affected by the presence or absence of particular examination findings.[5] This requires specific studies to determine the likelihood ratio of the diagnosis given the presence or absence of the clinical sign. The use of likelihood ratios in physical examination has recently been reviewed.[4] If there is more than one clinical finding, the likelihood ratios can *only* be combined if the findings are independent.[5]

When this has previously been studied, clinical prediction rules have sometimes been generated from the data (see Chapter 3).[4] Clearly, these studies have not been performed for every possible diagnosis and every possible clinical examination finding. Therefore, we can only appreciate the diagnostic value of certain physical examination findings in particular contexts, and the quality of the literature must also be considered. The take-home message, however, is to reflect on what is being examined and why, hone the skills necessary for proficient clinical examination and consider whether the findings are discriminatory and aid the diagnostic process.

INITIAL IMPRESSION

Some parts of the patient examination occur while taking the history. This has been referred to as the 'eyeball test' or 'end-of-bed-o-gram'.[6] For example, many non-verbal cues, such as how the patient is sitting, standing or lying, inform the initial assessment. These first impressions help a doctor answer the questions 'How sick is this patient?' and 'How quickly do I need to act?' An in-depth discussion on making these assessments is beyond the scope of this book. However, we point out that it is 'system 1 thinking' that often comes into play here to gain a fast, intuitive impression of a patient.[6] The key point is that reflective practice and extensive clinical experience can help doctors to gain more accurate first impressions, although they should always be wary of jumping to conclusions and should review the information collected before making decisions.

OBSERVATIONAL SKILLS AND VISUAL LITERACY

When medical students are learning how to examine the cardiovascular system, a stepwise head-to-toe approach is used. For example, start with the hands (looking for signs related to cardiovascular disease), move to take the pulse and blood pressure, look for clues in the face and look for the jugular venous pressure at the neck, and so on. This is a good way to learn a thorough, comprehensive, systems-based examination. However, one of the pitfalls of this way of learning can be that the clinician goes into autopilot while doing this and looks without seeing.

Over the last two decades, some medical schools have included courses that use the visual arts to develop and guide observational skills and 'visual thinking strategies'.[7] Visual thinking strategies are used in a variety of fields. In medicine, 'visual literacy' is the ability to use visual clues in the clinical reasoning process.[8] Some medical courses have combined art sessions with didactic teaching on examination techniques. For example, at Harvard medical school, lectures have incorporated discussion of works of art with clinical examination and included 'Line and symmetry in the cranial nerve examination' and 'Texture and pattern recognition in the dermatologic examination'.[8] It is purported that such courses increase analytical thinking through the practising of appreciating works of art, which is enhanced with peer to peer discussion.[9] Alongside qualitative research, quantitative studies demonstrating that these courses have a positive impact (in terms of encouraging observational skills) are also emerging, although there are limitations and further research is needed.[8]

Practising the art of 'careful looking' so that visual information can be accurately described and interpreted is an extremely useful skill across the spectrum of medical and surgical specialties.[7] The term 'careful looking' is similar to the term 'active looking' (comprising unbiased inspection and accurate reporting), which has also been coined in this context.[8] We hope that this book and this chapter in particular will contribute to the practising of 'careful looking'.

USING THE HAND PHOTOGRAPHS IN THIS BOOK TO HELP DEVELOP OBSERVATIONAL SKILLS AND VISUAL LITERACY

In addition to demonstrating the various diagnostic strategies, the photographs of hands in this book can be used to develop observational skills and visual thinking strategies. When examining a patient, the first observations are often made from inspection of a patient's hands. There can be a multitude of signs in the hands relating to a plethora of conditions affecting all systems of the body. Signs in the hands can act as a signpost for what a clinician might expect to find when examining the rest of the patient. For example, the patient with a Z-thumb and swan neck deformity of the fingers suggests a diagnosis of rheumatoid arthritis, and one may then find fibrotic lungs, rheumatoid nodules, keratoconjunctivitis sicca, carpal tunnel syndrome and the effects of systemic inflammation. Alongside signs of pathology, a wealth of other observations can be made by inspection of a patient's hands (*Table 5.1*).

Table 5.1 Observations made on inspection of the hands

Question	Example findings
How old is the patient?	A rough estimate can be made by looking at the hands and condition of the skin
What sort of work might they do?	Does their skin condition suggest that they wash their hands frequently or work outdoors or in a predominantly manual role?
Do they wear any jewellery?	Could this be a source of allergy? Does it point towards marital status?
Are they anxious?	Anxiety can manifest as sweating and nail biting or skin picking
Do they have a tremor?	For example, is there a benign essential tremor or the pill rolling tremor of Parkinsonism?
What is the condition of the skin? Does it reveal any dermatological pathology?	Is the skin excessively dry? Is dermatitis or psoriasis present, for example? Is there evidence of sun damage (e.g. actinic keratoses or solar lentigos)?
Are there any colour changes in the skin? Do they have tattoos?	Slate grey skin may relate to amiodarone therapy, pigmented palmar creases can be seen in Addison's disease, very tanned hands can be seen in haemochromatosis, and white patches might indicate vitiligo. With tattoos, think about the possibility of blood-borne infections
What is the condition of the nails?	Look for signs such as tar-stained nails of a heavy smoker, spoon-shaped nails (koilonychia) relating to iron deficiency, leukonychia (liver disease) and pitting and ridging (psoriasis)
Are there any potential pathological signs in the nails?	Are there, for example, splinter haemorrhages (endocarditis), nail fold infarcts (vasculitis) or clubbing?
Does the patient have a musculoskeletal or neurological condition?	Look, for example, for muscle wasting, signs of rheumatoid arthritis, claw hand from ulnar nerve damage and osteoarthritis
Has the patient had a previous hand surgery?	Look for surgical scars relating to joint replacements, carpal tunnel release and trauma, for example
Are the hands well perfused?	Look for pallor and, on examination, temperature and capillary refill time

Look at this patient's hands (Figure 5.1). What observations can you make?

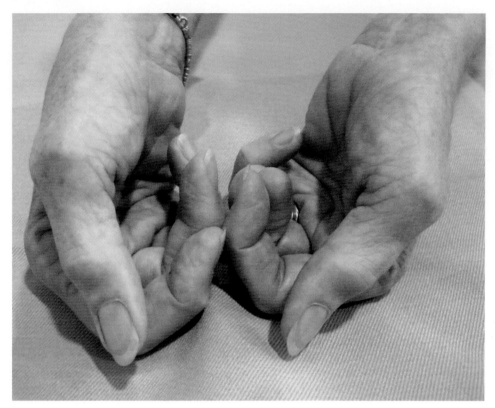

Fig. 5.1 The patient's hands.

Suggested observations are as follows:

- The patient is white and probably female.
- They are wearing jewellery on the ring finger of the left hand and a bracelet at the right wrist.
- The nails are manicured and in good condition.
- There are solar lentigos/freckles on the right hand.
- On the left hand, the middle and ring fingers are incomplete (note – from the patient's history, this was due to traumatic amputation).

A NOTE ON SKIN EXAMINATION

The cases in this book are based on clinical signs in the hands. Hence it is pertinent to include a brief note regarding the examination of the skin as it is relevant to many of the cases that follow.

The British Association of Dermatologists (BAD) has produced a useful guide for medical students and junior doctors for examining the skin.[10] The guide suggests following an 'Inspect, describe, palpate, systematic check' routine. First, inspect to gain a general impression of the extent and distribution of any lesions. The BAD suggests using the SCAM mnemonic to describe lesions:

- Size.
- Shape.
- Colour.
- Associated secondary change.
- Morphology.
- Margin.

In addition, the BAD suggests the ABCD mnemonic for pigmented lesions:

- Asymmetry.
- Irregular Border.
- Two or more Colours present.
- Diameter >6 mm.[10]

Next, palpate the lesion and describe what you feel. For example, is the skin rough or smooth? Is it thickened or lichenified? Finally, also examine the hair and scalp, nails and mucous membranes and any other body systems that may have related pathology (e.g. consider examining the chest of a patient with systemic sclerosis).

A 68-year-old retired painter and decorator presents in primary care with a long-standing (more than 8-week history) cough. He is a lifelong non-smoker. His past medical history includes hypertension and hypercholesterolaemia, and he takes a beta-blocker and a statin.

1 What might be the differential diagnosis for a long-standing cough?

A suggested differential diagnosis might include:

- Upper airway cough syndrome (includes postnasal drip).
- Gastro-oesophageal reflux.
- Bronchitis.
- Side-effect of angiotensin-converting enzyme inhibitors.
- Infections such as pneumonia, tuberculosis and *Bordetella pertussis*.
- Endobronchial tumours, bronchiectasis and interstitial lung disease, which are less common causes in primary care (although cough is the most common symptom of lung cancer).

A careful history reveals that the patient has felt short of breath when going for long walks or going upstairs; otherwise there are no additional features.

2 You decide to examine the patient for signs of respiratory disease and start with his hands. Both show the same signs. What do you notice in Figure 5.2?

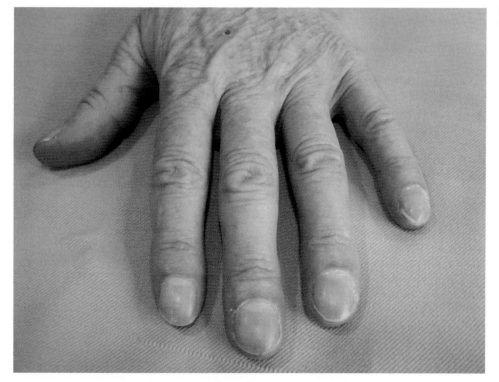

Fig. 5.2 The patient's left hand.

This is the left hand of an older white man. There are prominent veins over the dorsum of the hand and what looks like a scab. Clubbing is present in the fingernails.

3 What pattern of features can be used to identify clubbing as a clinical sign?

Features in the nails consistent with clubbing are:

- Schamroth's sign: when the dorsal surfaces of the terminal phalanges of the fingers are opposed, a diamond-shaped window should be seen, but this is absent in clubbing. However, evidence in the literature for the reliability of this sign is lacking.[11]
- Periungual oedema with softening of the nail bed.[12]
- A greater than 180° angle between the proximal nail fold and the nail bed (the Lovibond angle).[12]

4 What else might you want to find out regarding these nail changes?

Factors to consider include:

- Is the problem bilateral?
- Does it also affect the toes?
- How, if at all, has the patient been affected by this problem?

Clubbing is a clinical sign (not a diagnosis) and it is important to investigate further to establish a possible cause. Hence questions related to possible causes of these nail changes might include whether any other family members are affected (is it the hereditary form of clubbing rather than the form that indicates pathology?) and whether there are any changes in bowel habit (thinking of inflammatory bowel disease, for example) or other symptoms relevant to the presence of clubbing.

5 Complete *Table 5.2* to categorise the possible causes of clubbing by system of the body.

Table 5.2 Causes of clubbing

System	Clubbing may be a clinical manifestation of the following diagnoses
Cardiovascular	
Respiratory	
Gastrointestinal	
Congenital/familial	
Chronic infection	

Table 5.3 shows the completed table.

In this case, the patient was initially referred for a chest X-ray, which showed reticular shadowing predominantly in the lower zones. Lung function tests revealed a restrictive defect, and the diagnosis of idiopathic fibrosing alveolitis was confirmed by high-resolution CT.

Table 5.3 Completed table of causes of clubbing

System	Clubbing may be a clinical manifestation of the following conditions (not an exhaustive list)
Cardiovascular	• Cyanotic congenital cardiac disease • Infective endocarditis • Atrial myxoma
Respiratory	• Cystic fibrosis, Kartagener's disease • Fibrosing alveolitis • Bronchiectasis • Pulmonary tuberculosis • Lung malignancy, especially small cell lung cancer
Gastrointestinal	• Inflammatory bowel disease: Crohn's disease and ulcerative colitis • Malabsorption, e.g. coeliac disease • Chronic liver disease
Congenital/ familial	• Primary hypertrophic osteoarthropathy
Chronic infection	• HIV

This case follows the 'inspect, describe, palpate, systematic check format' and starts with a general inspection. The patient is a 61-year-old man.

1 Look at the hands in Figures 5.3 and 5.4. What observations can you make?

Fig. 5.3 The hands of the 61-year-old man.

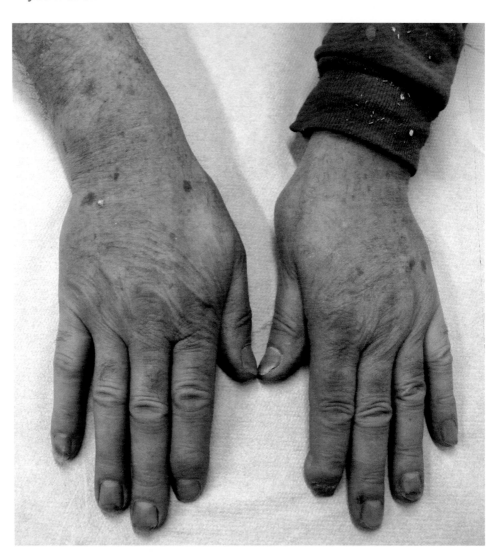

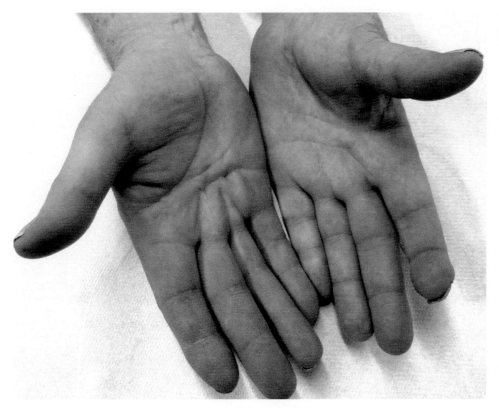

Fig. 5.4 The palmar aspect of the patient's hands.

These are the hands of a middle-aged man. The skin looks tanned and there are a few solar lentigos on each hand. From the clothing, it looks like this man may work in the construction industry or does DIY. The nails do not look to be in good condition (this is discussed in more detail later in the case). At the right wrist and forearm, there are several flat, pink lesions (discussed later). On the dorsum of the right hand, there is a small white scaly papule. From these images, it is not possible to tell if the lesions are bilateral.

There are no lesions on the palmar aspect of the hands. The skin is dry but in good condition. The palmar fascia looks thickened close to the middle and ring fingers on the right hand, and this is consistent with early Dupuytren's contracture (see Chapter 6). There is a fixed flexion deformity of the left distal interphalangeal joint and the left index finger has lost its tip.

2 Look more closely at the forearm. How would you describe the lesions shown in Figures 5.5 and 5.6?

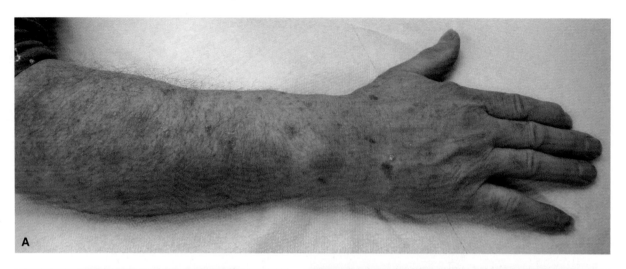

A

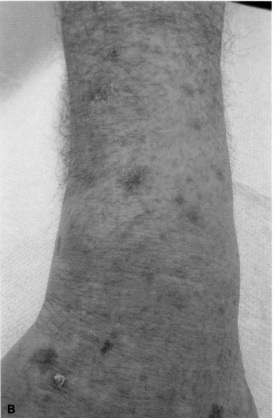

B

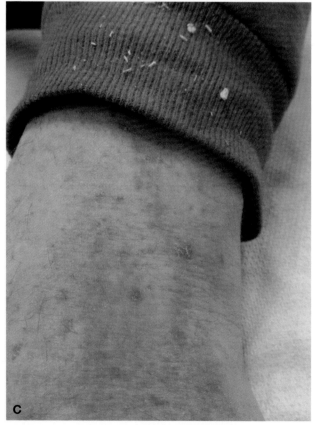

C

Fig. 5.5A–C The patient's skin.

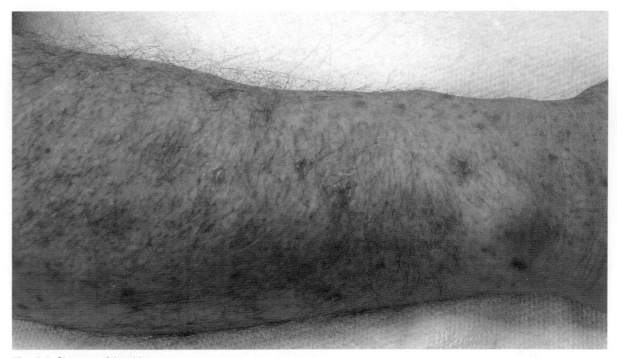

Fig. 5.6 Close-up of the skin.

Remember the SCAM mnemonic. These lesions can be described as a rash as they are widespread. They are distributed over the extensor surface of the forearm and wrist. There are several circular (approximately 1 cm diameter), pink, scaly plaques on the forearm. At the wrist is a white, scaly papule approximately 0.5 cm in size. At the patient's left wrist there are further pink, scaly papules, indicating that the condition is bilateral.

3 What is your differential diagnosis on the basis that these are long-standing lesions?

The differential diagnosis for the lesions include eczema, psoriasis, tinea infection, pityriasis rosea and actinic keratoses.

The patient admits to scratching the scale off the lesions on the forearm. On palpation, these lesions are rough and slightly elevated.

4 As part of the systematic check, you look more closely at the patient's nails. What features are present in Figures 5.7–5.10?

Fig. 5.7 The fingernails on the right hand.

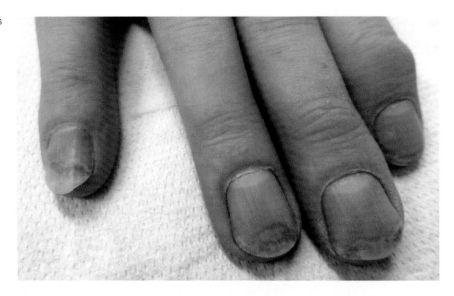

Fig. 5.8 The left hand.

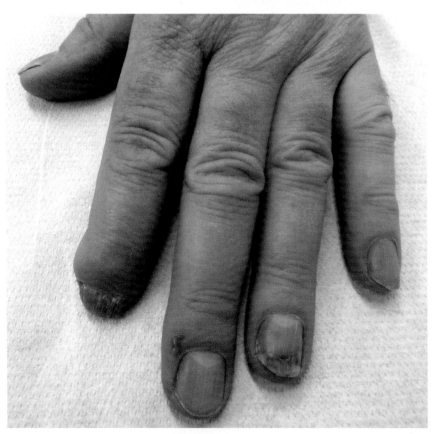

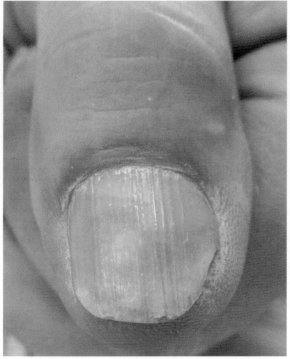

Fig.5.9 The thumb on the left hand.   **Fig.5.10** The forefinger on the left hand.

The features of note are the presence of pitting, vertical ridging and onycholysis. Onycholysis refers to the separation of the distal nail plate from the nail bed.[10]

The forefinger on the left hand has undergone previous trauma to the distal phalanx. There is widespread vertical ridging and a green colour to the nail indicating possible *Pseudomonas* infection.

5 Given the presence of the nail features, can you make a diagnosis?

The patient has psoriasis with nail involvement. Psoriasis is the most common skin disease that affects the nails, and 50% of patients with psoriasis have nail involvement.[13] Of those with psoriasis, 10–30% will develop psoriatic arthropathy.[14] Those patients with psoriatic arthropathy are more likely to have nail changes.[10] Nail changes are a poor prognostic factor for psoriasis.[13]

6 What else might you consider examining in this patient?

Psoriasis more commonly affects the fingernails but it would be useful to check whether the toenails are also affected. You could examine the scalp, umbilicus and behind the ears to look for psoriasis in these areas. In addition, an examination of the joints might reveal psoriatic arthropathy.

7 What other signs might you see on examination that are typical of psoriasis?

Psoriasis demonstrates Köbnerisation (plaques can be seen in areas of previous trauma or scarring). In addition, when the scaly top of a plaque is scratched off, capillary bleeding is revealed (Auspitz sign).[10]

The onycholysis in this patient's nails is very striking.

8 What is the pathological process behind this phenomenon?

Psoriatic plaques can be present in the distal nail matrix and the nail bed. Here they are referred to as salmon or oil spots.[13] When these plaques reach the hyponychium (the epithelium that is underlying the free edge of the nail), they cause the nail to come away from the nail bed; this is referred to as onycholysis.[13]

9 The patient is worried about psoriatic arthropathy and asks you about this. What features would you ask about or look for?

We know that this patient already has skin psoriasis with nail involvement. Note that individuals with nail changes have an increased risk of developing psoriatic arthropathy.

Ask about and look for:

- Dactylitis (swelling of the digit).
- Joint swelling (a key distinguisher from rheumatoid arthritis is involvement of the distal interphalangeal joints).[14]
- Pain in the heel (which may suggest Achilles enthesitis) – enthesitis is a key feature in psoriatic arthritis.

The diagnosis of psoriatic arthritis is largely clinical. The presence of a negative test for rheumatoid factor helps to point towards the diagnosis and this feature is included in the CASPAR criteria for diagnosing psoriatic arthritis.[14] In terms of radiographical evidence, look at X-rays of the hands and feet for juxta-articular new bone formation.[14]

A 58-year-old retail assistant has mild iron deficiency anaemia. This is a long-standing problem attributed to frequent nose bleeds. She suffered a gastrointestinal bleed 10 years ago. She takes iron tablets regularly but no other medication.

1 What might be possible causes for frequent epistaxis?

- Dry nasal membranes.
- Anticoagulants such as apixaban and warfarin.
- Coagulopathies such as von Willebrand's disease and haemophilia.
- Irritants to the nose.

2 What do you observe about the patient's lower face (Figures 5.11 and 5.12)?

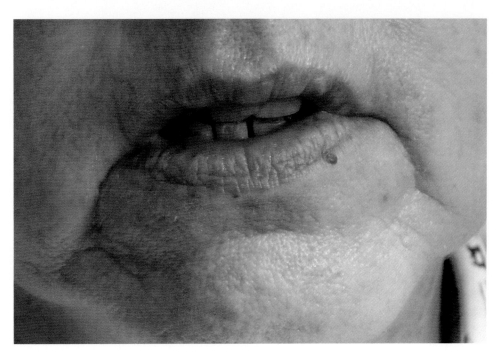

Fig. 5.11 The patient's lower face.

Fig. 5.12 The patient's
mouth.

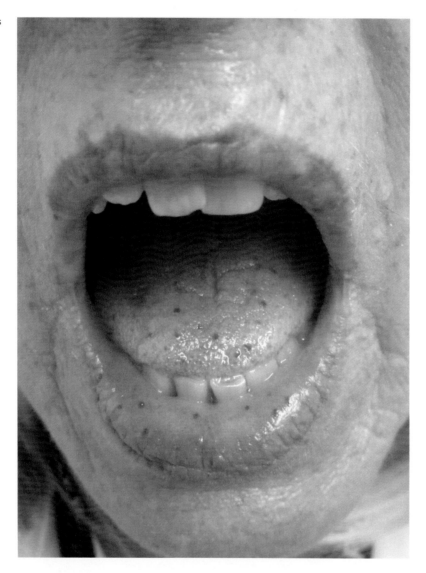

From the photographs, the skin looks in good condition. The dentition looks good from what
can be seen of the teeth. This patient has perioral telangiectasia and telangiectasia on the lips
and tongue.

3 What do you notice about the patient's hands (Figures 5.13 and 5.14)?

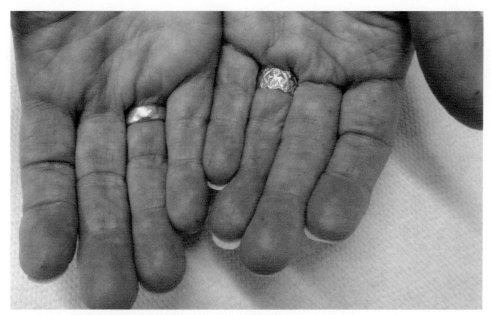

Fig. 5.13 The patient's hands.

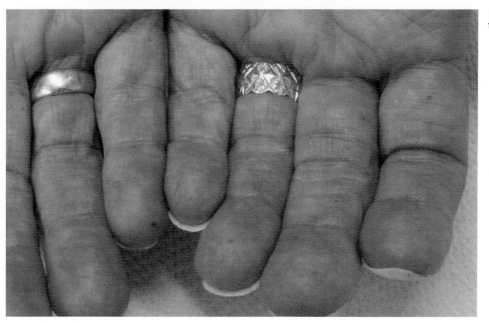

Fig. 5.14 Close-up of the fingers.

The skin on the palmar aspects of this woman's hands is in good condition. She wears jewellery on the ring fingers of both hands. There are telangiectases on the fingers of both hands.

Note: a telangiectasia occurs from a direct connection between an arteriole and a vein (bypassing capillaries) and appears on a mucocutaneous surface.[15]

4 Is there a unifying diagnosis that might fit with a history of frequent nose bleeds, anaemia and perioral and palmar telangiectasia?

Hereditary haemorrhagic telangiectasia (HHT; also known as Osler–Weber–Rendu syndrome) is an autosomal dominantly inherited disease in which multiple telangiectasia and arterio-venous malformations (AVMs) form. This can lead to epistaxis and iron deficiency anaemia, gastrointestinal bleeding and stroke.[15] Liver failure and high-output heart failure can result from hepatic and pulmonary AVMs, and brain abscesses can occur due to passage of bacteria via right-to-left shunts from pulmonary AVMs.[15] The recurrent epistaxis is a hallmark of this disease as 50% of patients have epistaxis by age 10 years, and 95% will develop recurrent epistaxis over the course of their lives.[16]

The diagnosis of HHT is largely clinical, although the genetic mutation responsible can often be identified. The Curaçao criteria (where HHT is diagnosed if three out of four are present) are used for diagnosis.[17] These criteria look for the presence of:

- Spontaneous and recurrent epistaxis.
- Cutaneo-mucous telangiectasia.
- Visceral lesions.
- A positive family history.

5 Does this patient fit the diagnostic criteria for this condition?

Given the history of a previous gastrointestinal bleed, the cutaneo-mucous telangiectasia and the history of recurrent epistaxis, this patient does fit the diagnostic criteria for HHT.

6 Where else might you find telangiectasia on examination of this patient?

Remember that the telangiectasia are cutaneo-mucous in nature and hence a full examination of the skin may reveal telangiectasia elsewhere (**Figure 5.15**).

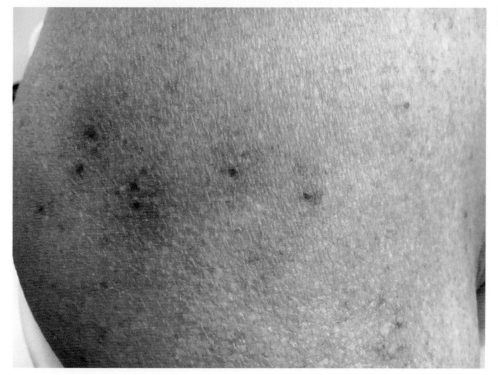

Fig. 5.15 Skin on the upper arm.

DIAGNOSING RARE DISEASES

Patients who have a rare disease can be subject to diagnostic delay.[18] Evans encourages clinicians to 'dare to think rare' in the context of patients in whom patterns emerge that are divergent from the norm.[19] The key skill in primary care is not to know all the clinical presentations for the vast number of rare diseases, but to identify patients who have persistent problems for which we have been unable to provide a satisfactory explanation and to take a whole-person approach, coordinating effectively with specialists to arrive at a diagnosis.

Just as other medical students have practised the art of 'careful looking' via the keen observation of fine art, in this final case we present a brief case involving the hands of a 71-year-old man. This case is predominantly a visual case, not to highlight pattern recognition but to encourage the reader to look for detail in all the images that follow.

1 **First, make as many observations as you can about the dorsal and palmar aspects of the hands in Figures 5.16 and 5.17**

Fig. 5.16 The dorsal aspects of the hands.

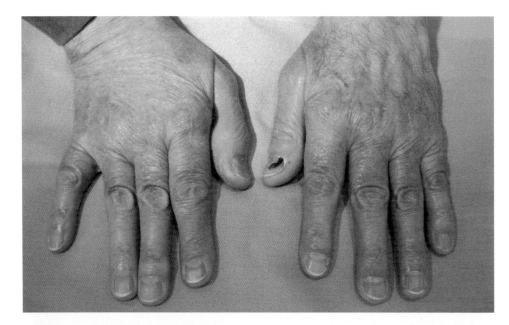

Fig. 5.17 The palmar aspects of the hands.

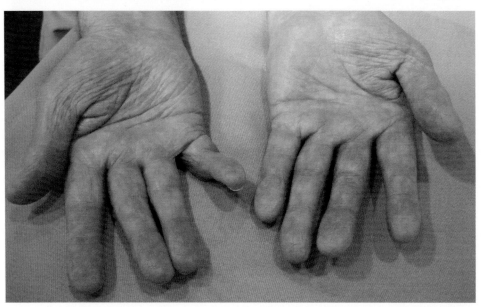

These are the hands of an older white man. The cuff of a grey jumper is just visible. The skin and nails appear to be in good condition apart from a red-brown lesion in the left thumbnail that comprises approximately one third of the nail plate. The nails are neatly trimmed. There is light brown hair over the back of both hands, and some of the veins are visible. There is wasting of the thenar eminences bilaterally, and an ulnar deviation flexion deformity of the right little finger.

2 What might the red-brown lesion in the thumbnail be in Figure 5.18?

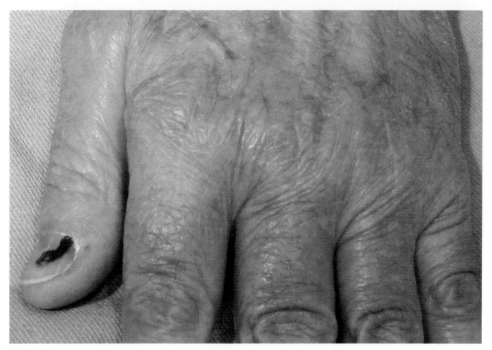

Fig. 5.18 Close-up of the dorsal aspect of the left hand.

This is likely to be a subungal haematoma secondary to trauma but the possibility of melanoma should be considered.

In close-up, some vertical scars are just visible over the metacarpophalangeal joints of the fingers of each hand.

3 From the observations you have made of the hands, what do you suspect the overall diagnosis is?

This patient has rheumatoid arthritis and has undergone multiple metacarpophalangeal joint arthroplasties.

4 Figures 5.19–5.21 show the left hand before and after the surgery. What is the most striking feature in the left hand prior to surgery (Figure 5.19)?

Fig. 5.19 The left hand before surgery.

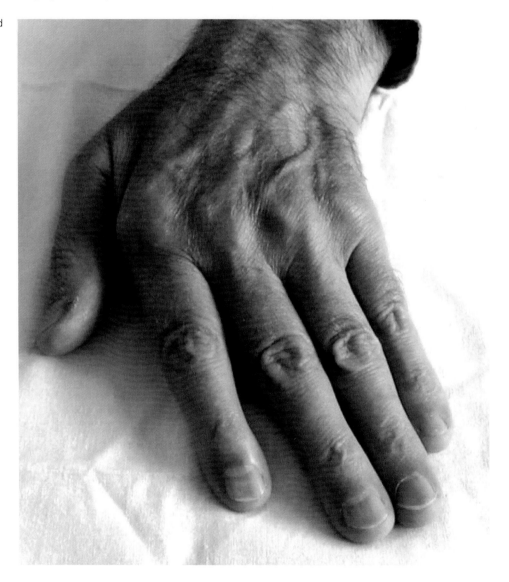

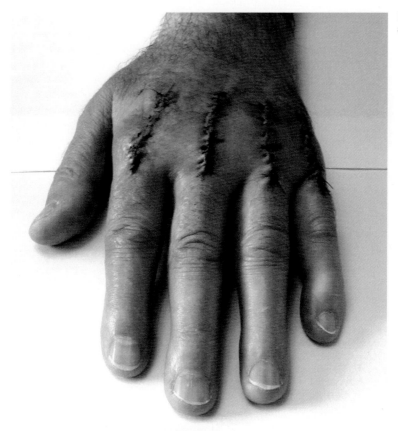

Fig. 5.20 The left hand after surgery.

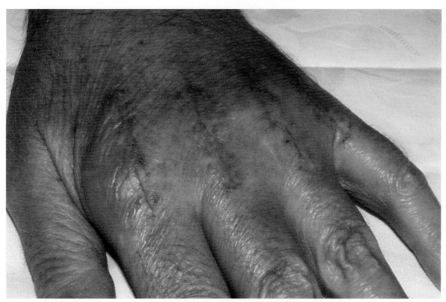

Fig. 5.21 The left hand with healing of the incision sites.

The most striking feature is the ulnar deviation of the metacarpophalangeal joints.
(We thank the patient who kindly provided pictures from his own collection.)

SUMMARY

- This chapter briefly describes evidence-based examination, initial impressions, observational skills and visual literacy.
- It explains how the hand photographs in this book can be used to help develop the art of 'careful looking', and the approach to dermatological examination is described.
- Four cases are explored with an emphasis on keen observation. These patients demonstrate clubbing, psoriasis with nail involvement, hereditary haemorrhagic telangectasia and joint replacement secondary to rheumatoid arthritis.

REFERENCES

1 Elder AT, McManus IC, Patrick A, Nair K, Vaughan L, Dacre J. The value of the physical examination in clinical practice: an international survey. *Clin Med* 2017;**17**:490–8.

2 Mohammed KA. Clinical examination nowadays. *Lancet* 2016;**388**:559–60.

3 Feddock CA. The lost art of clinical skills. *Am J Med* 2007;**120**:374–8.

4 Garibaldi BT, Olson APJ. The hypothesis-driven physical examination. *Med Clin N Am* 2018;**102**:433–42.

5 Cooper N, Frain J. *The ABC of Clinical Reasoning*. Chichester: Wiley Blackwell; 2017.

6 Adams E, Goyder C, Heneghan C, Brand L, Aijawi R. Clinical reasoning of junior doctors in emergency medicine: a grounded theory study. *Emerg Med J* 2017;**34**:70–5.

7 Russell SW. Improving observational skills to enhance the clinical examination. *Med Clin N Am* 2018;**102**:495–507.

8 Naghshineh S, Hafler JP, Miller AR, *et al*. Formal art observation training improves medical students' visual diagnostic skills. *J Gen Int Med* 2008;**23**:991–7.

9 Reilly JM, Ring J, Duke L. Visual thinking strategies: a new role for art in medical education. *Fam Med* 2005;**37**:250–2.

10 Yi Zhen Chiang N, Verbov J. *Dermatology: A Handbook for Medical Students and Junior Doctors*. London: British Association of Dermatologists.

11 Sarkar M, Mahesh D, Madabhavi I. Digital clubbing. *Lung India* 2012;**29**:354–62.

12 Rutherford JD. Digital clubbing. *Circulation* 2013;**127**:1997–9.

13 Haneke E. Nail psoriasis: clinical features, pathogenesis, differential diagnoses, and management. *Psoriasis (Auckl)* 2017;**7**:51–63.

14 Lenman M, Abraham S. Diagnosis and management of psoriatic arthropathy in primary care. *Br J Gen Pract* 2014;**64**:424–5.

15 Topical corticosteroids. 2018. Available from https://www.nhs.uk/conditions/topical-steroids/.

16 Kritharis A, Al-Samkari H, Kuter DJ. Hereditary hemorrhagic telangiectasia: diagnosis and management from the hematologist's perspective. *Haematologica* 2018;**103**:1433–43.

17 Grigg C, Anderson D, Earnshaw J. Diagnosis and treatment of hereditary hemorrhagic telangiectasia. *Ochsner J* 2017;**17**:157–61.

18 Schieppati A, Henter J-I, Daina E, Aperia A. Why rare diseases are an important medical and social issue. *Lancet* 2008;**371**:2039–41.

19 Evans WRH. Dare to think rare: diagnostic delay and rare diseases. *Br J Gen Pract* 2018;**68**:224.

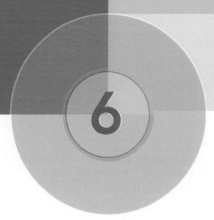

Spot diagnosis and
pattern recognition

6

INTRODUCTION

Pattern recognition is the starting point for generating a list of differential diagnoses that can then be tested. It is a form of non-analytic reasoning in which a clinician forms an unconscious link between a previously remembered clinical presentation and their current patient.[1] Heneghan *et al.* refer to it as 'pattern recognition trigger', whereby, in the initial stages, a particular pattern triggers the need to collect further information and refine a hypothesis.[2] Thus, non-analytic and analytic reasoning are combined. Pattern recognition is also used in the refinement stage ('pattern recognition fit'), in which the signs and symptoms are recognised as fitting a pattern of disease known to the clinician, and a diagnosis is made.[2]

This differs from a 'spot diagnosis', which occurs when a clinical presentation is quickly recognised and a single diagnosis is reached there and then without prior data gathering. A spot diagnosis can be reached instantly by reacting to an auditory or visual cue from the patient, such as recognising a cold sore.[2] They rely on multiple clinical experiences of cases of the particular disease, often based on visual memory. In the study by Heneghan *et al.*, established GPs were found to use the spot diagnosis strategy in 20% of their cases.[2]

Recent work in primary care has revealed that experienced GPs tend to use pattern recognition frequently in their clinical reasoning.[3] Clinicians develop pattern recognition with increasing levels of experience but the key word here is *experience*. Pattern recognition works best when a clinician has seen multiple similar cases that are presenting with a similar, recognisable pattern. The downside of this strategy is that it can fail when there is an atypical presentation of a problem.[3]

DANGERS OF SPOT DIAGNOSIS AND PATTERN RECOGNITION

Spot diagnosis and pattern recognition can lure clinicians into taking shortcuts. The key is to always fully review your findings in the context of the patient. Using pattern recognition alone can lead to error but using it alongside analytical approaches helps reduce diagnostic error.[1] Since pattern recognition is rapid and intuitive, it can lead to error by premature closure and hence it is wise to confirm a diagnosis by seeking further evidence. Studies have shown that analytic reasoning alone is not necessarily superior but a combined approach yields the best results.[4]

CASES IN THIS CHAPTER

Look at the patients in Cases 6.1 and 6.2 and make a *spot* diagnosis. These cases test your powers of observation as patients can have multiple connected or unconnected pathologies for which visual clues can be sought.

In Case 6.3, look carefully at this patient's hands; do you recognise a pattern to the signs, and if so what is your differential diagnosis? Think about what the problem might be and generate a working diagnosis. Next, think about other features of this disease that you could look for or ask about to confirm your hypothesis.

You examine the hands of a 75-year-old man who complains of progressive deformity of his hands (**Figures 6.1–6.3**).

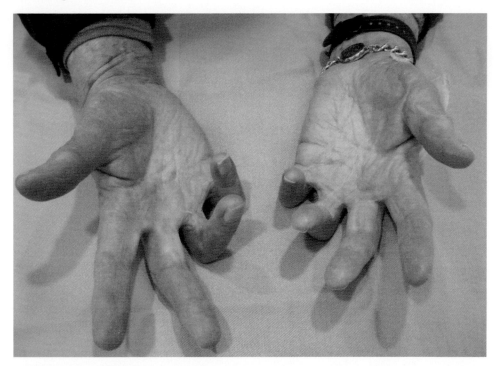

Fig. 6.1 The hands of the 75-year-old man.

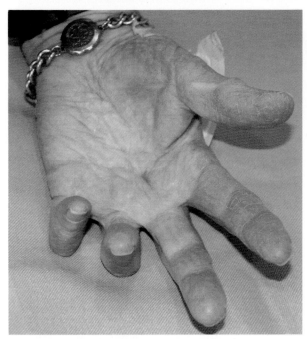

Fig. 6.2 The patient's left hand.

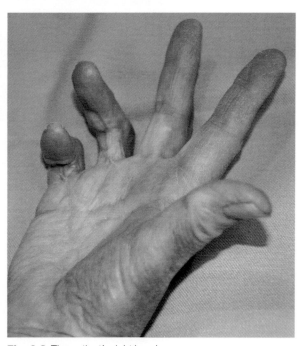

Fig. 6.3 The patient's right hand.

1 What is the diagnosis?

The diagnosis is Dupuytren's contracture.

2 What features are shown in these hands that lead you to this diagnosis?

The features are shown more closely in **Figures 6.4–6.6**.

Fig. 6.4 Thickening of the palmar fascia revealing a visible cord of thickened fascia.

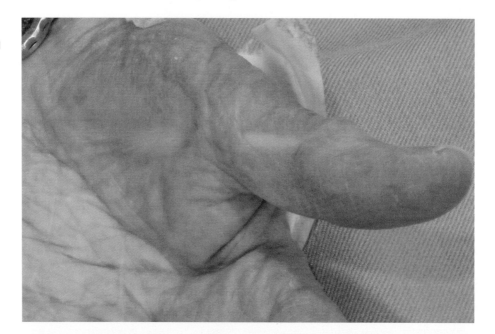

Fig. 6.5 Fixed flexion deformity (contracture) of the fingers.

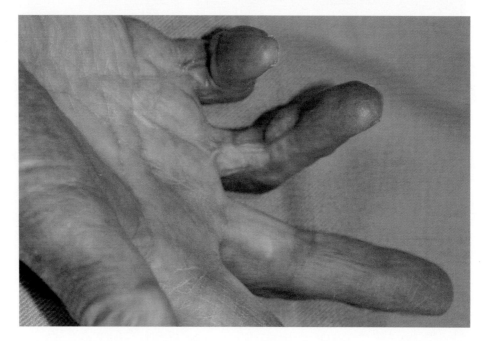

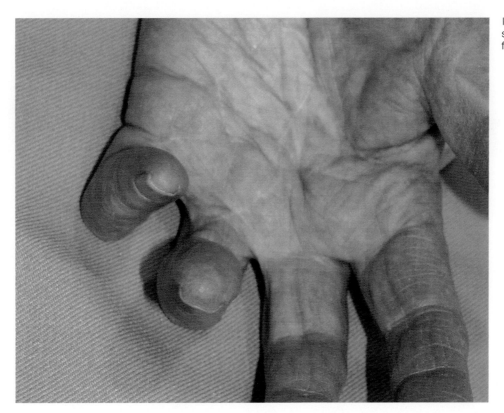

Fig. 6.6 Surgical scars from previous fasciectomies.

3 What might you ask about in the history to determine whether this patient has any factors that are associated with this problem?

Dupuytren's contracture typically affects men and is bilateral in 40% of patients.[5] Positive family history, alcoholic liver disease, Peyronie's disease, diabetes mellitus, smoking and possibly anticonvulsants are associated with the condition. This is an area of ongoing research; for example, a recent study has shown an association with vibration transfer from the long-term operation of vibrating tools.[6]

4 What other notable features are there in the photos?

Other notable features in this patient are as follows:

- The condition is bilateral and this patient has a medical alert bracelet on his left wrist.
- The patient has features of Dupuytren's disease with scars from previous surgery. Recurrence of the disease is common.[7]

A NOTE ABOUT PATHOPHYSIOLOGY

Research continues into the mechanisms that underlie this condition but it is known that myofibroblast proliferation and collagen deposition play a major role. The palmar fascial bands change to become nodules and cords as a result.[7]

5 Why might a patient with this diagnosis wear a medical alert bracelet (Figure 6.7)?

Fig. 6.7 Patient medical alert bracelet.

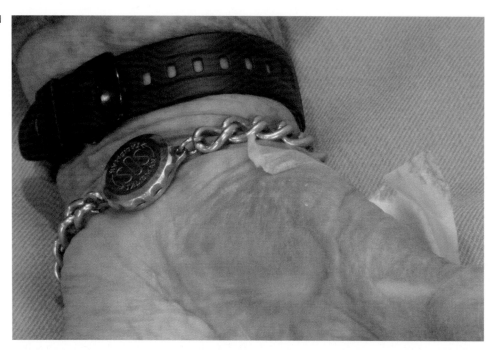

As discussed above, Dupuytren's contractures can be associated with long-term conditions. A patient with insulin-dependent diabetes or an individual who has had a liver transplant (e.g. due to alcoholic liver disease) may choose to wear such a bracelet.

A 74-year-old woman presents because the middle finger on her left hand is locking in the position shown in **Figure 6.8**.

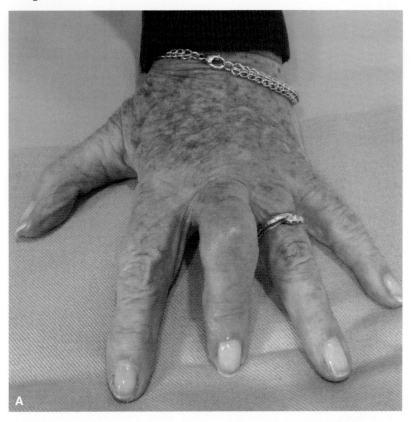

Fig. 6.8A, B
The patient's left hand.

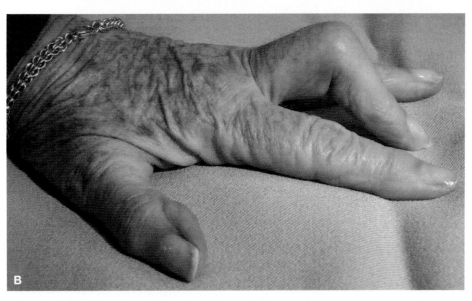

To straighten the finger she has to manipulate it with her other hand (**Figure 6.9**).

Fig. 6.9 The patient straightens the middle finger.

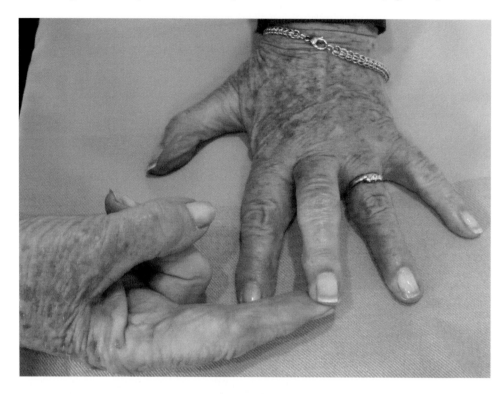

1 Describe the deformity in this patient's left hand.

There is a fixed flexion deformity of the proximal interphalangeal joint of the middle finger of the left hand.

2 Can this condition be recognised as a spot diagnosis? If so, what is it?

When seeing this patient's problem, we can instantly recognise it as trigger finger (also known as stenosing tenosynovitis) if we have seen it before.

3 What other symptoms might you ask about in the history?

Other symptoms you could ask about are:

- Painful clicking on flexing and extending the digit.
- Pain at the base of the digit or in the palm.
- Stiffness when moving the digit.

4 Which clinicians are most likely to encounter patients with this condition?

Clinicians likely to encounter this condition include hand surgeons, GPs, rheumatologists and endocrinologists.[8]

A NOTE ABOUT PATHOPHYSIOLOGY

In trigger finger, there is reduced space for the flexor tendon through the A1 pulley system, which may be caused by pulley hypertrophy, fibrocartilaginous metaplasia or inflammation of the flexor tendon or sheath.[8] This lack of space causes the symptoms of trigger finger.

Conditions associated with this condition include diabetes mellitus, rheumatoid arthritis, gout, hypothyroidism, carpal tunnel syndrome and Dupuytren's contracture.[8]

HOW CAN THE CONDITION BE TREATED?

The HANDGUIDE study was published in 2014 and aimed to provide some consensus guidelines on how trigger finger (among other common hand conditions) should be treated based on the current evidence and the opinion of experts in the field.[9] The consensus was that there were broadly four options, which could be placed in a hierarchy: splinting, corticosteroid injections, corticosteroid injections plus splinting, and hand surgery.[9] In primary care, corticosteroid injections can be tried, but it is important to remember that the digital nerves can run in close proximity to the A1 pulley so care needs to be taken when injecting.[8] Hand surgery involves trigger finger release, which has been quoted as having success rates of 90% – approximately the same as the success rate for corticosteroid injection.[8]

A 70-year-old woman complains of pain in her fingers. She has particularly noticed this when it is cold outside. She reports she has had stiffness in the fingers for a long time but now describes difficulty moving the little finger on her left hand.

1 What would you ask to explore further the problem she experiences with the cold?

You ask her what exactly happens to her hands when she goes out in the cold. She is able to give you a good description of fingers that become white, then blue and then very red, associated with pain. This pattern fits with the triphasic colour change associated with Raynaud's phenomenon (white due to ischaemia, blue from cyanosis and red from reactive hyperaemia). You might also ask her about smoking as this is a risk factor for Raynaud's phenomenon.

2 You examine her hands (Figures 6.10–6.12). Do you recognise a pattern from the history and photographs?

Fig. 6.10 The hands of the 70-year-old woman.

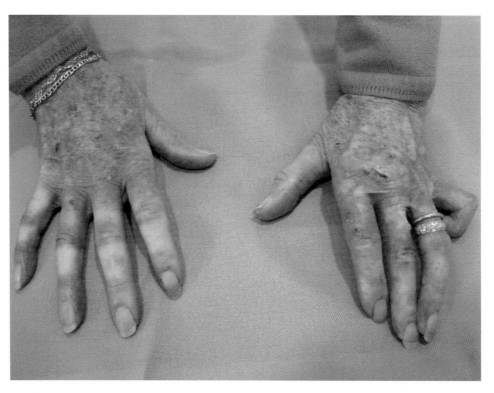

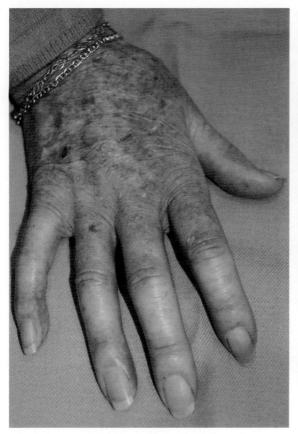

Fig. 6.11 The patient's right hand.

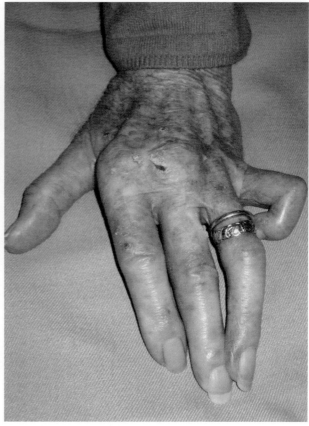

Fig. 6.12 The patient's left hand.

The history is consistent with Raynaud's phenomenon. In the photos, the prominent features are of tight, thickened, shiny, hairless skin with loss of skin creases (sclerodactyly) and joint deformity. Remember that the thickening and tightness of the skin is detected on palpation. This pattern of features coupled with the history of Raynaud's phenomenon would fit with scleroderma (note that at this stage, without examining the rest of the patient, we do not know if this represents limited or diffuse systemic sclerosis). Approximately 90% of patients with systemic sclerosis have Raynaud's phenomenon, so it is important to take a careful history in this respect.[10] In addition, approximately 95% of individuals with the diagnosis show signs of sclerodactyly.[10]

3 Figures 6.13 and 6.14 show a different patient with systemic sclerosis, demonstrating the deformity and sclerodactyly caused by this disease. What other features in the hands (not shown in this patient) might you find that would also be present in a patient with systemic sclerosis?

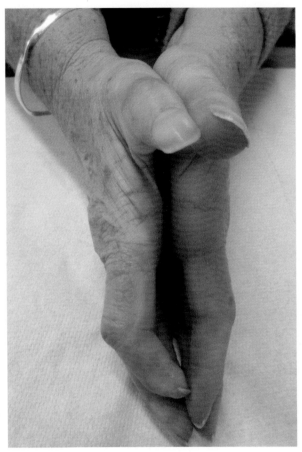

Fig. 6.13 Sclerodactyly and deformity.

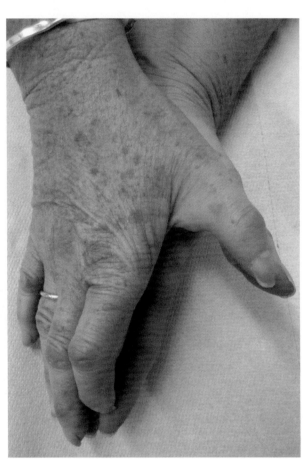

Fig. 6.14 Another view of the sclerodactyly and deformity in this patient.

In systemic sclerosis, you should look for telangiectases; these may occur on the palms (**Figure 16.15**), but are also very commonly found on the face. Note in **Figure 16.15** also the presence of coincidental 'avocado' hand (an injury caused by using a knife to remove an avocado stone).

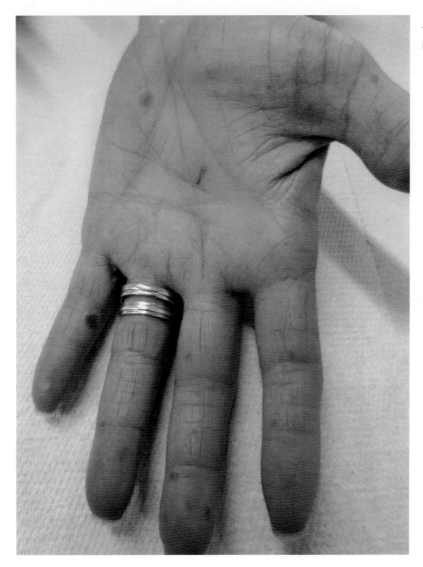

Fig. 6.15
Telangiectases of the palmar hand.

In addition, examine the nails folds for nail fold infarcts and look out for nail dystrophy. Calcinosis often occurs in the finger pulps (**Figure 6.16**). Also look for digital ulceration or evidence of past ulceration (**Figure 6.17**). With more advanced disease and severe sclerodactyly, there is often marked pulp atrophy, which tends to precede painful ulceration. There may also be hypo- or hyper-pigmented skin.

Fig. 6.16 Calcinosis of the finger pulp.

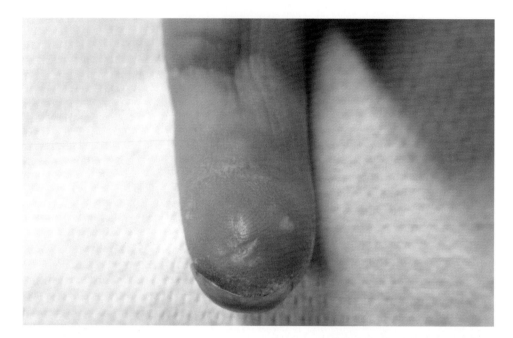

Fig. 6.17 A small area of previous ulceration that is healed at the base of the thumb.

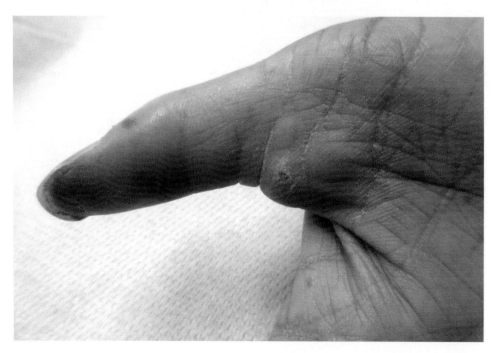

4 In the 70-year-old woman discussed above, you suspect systemic sclerosis. You examine her face (Figures 6.18 and 6.19). What characteristic changes in the mouth do you see?

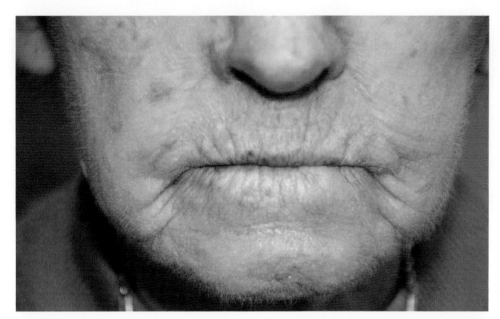

Fig. 6.18 The patient's closed mouth.

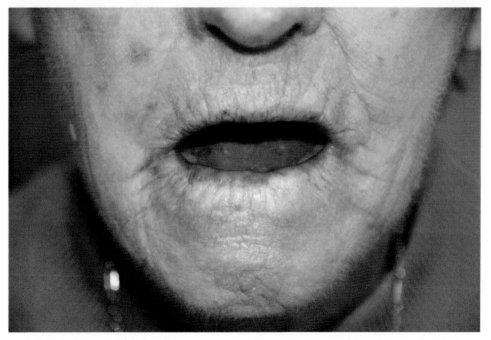

Fig. 6.19 The patient's open mouth.

These photographs show micostomia and tightening and puckering of the skin around the mouth. There are also telangiectases of the facial skin, lips and tongue.

5 On further exploring the history and on full examination of the patient, what might you expect to find (think in terms of body systems)?

Features of systemic sclerosis are shown in *Table 6.1*.

Table 6.1 Features of systemic sclerosis

System	Feature
General inspection	Weight loss
	Pinched nose
	Microstomia – limited opening of the mouth with surrounding skin puckering
Skin and nails	Sclerodermatous skin changes – oedematous, then indurated with loss of hair[11]
	Telangiectases
	Calcinosis
	Oedema
	Nails – disrupted capillary loops in the nail fold
Musculoskeletal	Arthralgia
	Joint stiffness
	Erosive arthritis – although it generally tends to be non-erosive unless there is an overlap
	Flexion contractures
Cardiovascular	Signs of myocarditis, pericarditis, pulmonary hypertension and restrictive cardiomyopathy
Respiratory	Fine end-inspiratory crackles indicating lung fibrosis
	Signs of pulmonary hypertension – cyanosis, right ventricular heave, loud pulmonary heart sound (P2), tricuspid regurgitation, peripheral oedema[11]
Gastrointestinal	Oesophageal dysmotility
	Other oesophageal problems such as strictures, reflux and dysphagia
	Intestinal dysmotility, which can lead to constipation
	Intestinal malabsorption, which can lead to steatorrhoea
Renal	Glomerulonephritis
	Malignant hypertension

SUMMARY

- This chapter explains two forms of non-analytic reasoning – pattern recognition and spot diagnosis – and considers the pitfalls of using strategies that rely on 'system 1 thinking'.
- The first two cases are discussed in the context of spot diagnosis.
- The final case, a patient with scleroderma, examines pattern recognition as a strategy.

REFERENCES

1 Pelaccia T, Tardif J, Triby E, Charlin B. An analysis of clinical reasoning through a recent and comprehensive approach: the dual-process theory. *Med Educ Online* 2011;**16**:5890–8.

2 Heneghan C, Glasziou P, Thompson M, *et al.* Diagnostic strategies used in primary care. *BMJ* 2009;**338**:b946.

3 Goyder CR, Jones CHD, Heneghan CJ, Thompson MJ. Missed opportunities for diagnosis: lessons learned from diagnostic errors in primary care. *Br J Gen Pract* 2015;**65**:e838–44.

4 Ark TK, Brooks LR, Eva KW. Giving learners the best of both worlds: do clinical teachers need to guard against teaching pattern recognition to novices? *Acad Med* 2006; **81**:405–9.

5 Hakim A, Clunie G, Haq I. *Oxford Handbook of Rheumatology*, 2nd ed. Oxford: Oxford University Press; 2008.

6 Descatha A, Carton M, Mediouni Z, *et al.* Association among work exposure, alcohol intake, smoking and Dupuytren's disease in a large cohort study (GAZEL). *BMJ Open* 2014;**4**:1–8.

7 van Dijk D, Finigan P, Gerber RA, Szczypa PP, Werker PMN. Recognition, diagnosis and referral of patients with Dupuytren's disease: a review of current concepts for general practitioners in Europe. *Curr Med Res Opin* 2013;**29**:269–77.

8 Akhtar S, Bradley MJ, Quinton DN, Burke FD. Management and referral for trigger finger/thumb. *BMJ* 2005;**331**:30–3.

9 Huisstede BMA, Hoogvliet P, Coert JH, Fridén J. Multidisciplinary consensus guideline for managing trigger finger: results from the European HANDGUIDE study. *Phys Ther* 2014;**94**:1421–33.

10 Young A, Khanna D. Systemic sclerosis: commonly asked questions by rheumatologists. *J Clin Rheum* 2015;**21**:149–55.

11 Kalra PA. *Essential Revision Notes for MRCP*, 3rd ed. Knutsford: Jaypee Brothers Medical Publishers.

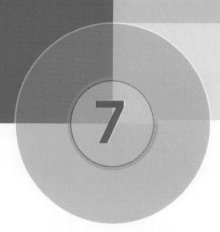

Red and yellow flags

7

INTRODUCTION

Red flags are signs or symptoms that are sought in the history or examination in order to consider serious conditions.[1] The presence of a red flag should trigger a detailed history, examination, further investigations and possible immediate treatment or referral to secondary care. Red flags serve as a method for clinicians to make sure they do not overlook a 'Do not miss' diagnosis such as cauda equina syndrome in a patient presenting with low back pain.[2]

Red flags can either be sought in a specific way (such as asking about dysphagia as a marker for oesophageal carcinoma) or in a general way by considering asking about the following red flags: fever and night sweats, unplanned weight loss, lumps, persistent pain and unusual bleeding.[3]

When patients present in primary care with symptoms such as low back pain, indigestion or headache, GPs will ask themselves, 'Does this symptom represent serious pathology that may require urgent referral such as admission to hospital or a "2-week wait" appointment to consider cancer?' Determining whether or not there are red flags related to the patient's presenting complaint can greatly assist in answering that question.

IDENTIFYING THE RED FLAGS FOR A PARTICULAR CONDITION

In general, red flags are listed in Clinical Knowledge Summaries (CKS) for given conditions and in national guidelines such as the National Institute for Health and Care Excellence (NICE) and Scottish Intercollegiate Guidelines Network (SIGN) guidelines. (CKS are produced on behalf of NICE to provide a concise, easily-accessible guide for primary care clinicians [https://cks.nice.org.uk/#?char=A].)

AVOIDING ERRORS

Sometimes it is not the signs or symptoms themselves that act as red flags but the circumstances surrounding the patient's presentation. For example, patients who repeatedly attend the emergency department with persistent symptoms, despite being previously investigated, could be considered a 'red flag' case, as can patients presenting on multiple occasions with the same symptoms to primary care. Errors may easily occur in their assessment due to anchoring (relying too heavily on the prior assessment of others) or factors such as the clinician's perception of the patient, which may adversely affect their judgement (in the above, for example, perhaps classifying these patients as 'frequent flyers', i.e. patients who tend to attend frequently but rarely have serious pathology).[4]

Use of red flag checklists is a good way to reduce error when taking a history, but Goyder *et al.* point out that the presenting complaint is sometimes itself a red flag, and even though it might be obvious, clinicians can sometimes fail to recognise this.[5]

YELLOW FLAGS

Determining the presence or absence of yellow flags is a diagnostic strategy aimed at influencing patient outcomes rather than arriving at a diagnostic label. The approach is an emerging one that is currently subject to research.

Yellow flags have previously been described as psychosocial factors that can indicate a risk of chronicity and disability.[6] However, more recently it has been suggested that the term should only relate to psychological risk factors for developing disability after musculoskeletal pain.[7] Most of the current literature details the use of yellow flags in the assessment and management of low back pain. Krismer and van Tulder suggest that yellow flags can indicate a less favourable and therefore chronic course of non-specific low back pain.[8]

Psychosocial yellow flags include individual factors such as obesity, smoking and low educational level, together with factors such as stress, anxiety and depression and occupational factors such as job dissatisfaction, monotony and poor work relations.[8] The psychological yellow flags have been grouped into beliefs and judgements (e.g. expecting the treatment not to work), emotional responses (e.g. anxiety) and pain behaviour (e.g. avoiding activities due to fear of pain).[7]

If we can identify the presence of yellow flags early, clinicians may have an opportunity to try to modify a patient's ideas and beliefs about a condition and/or refer for appropriate psychological therapies to try to prevent chronicity. In addition, clinicians may be able to help patients address certain yellow flags themselves, although some factors (e.g. social circumstances) may be more difficult to change.

Nicholas *et al.* conducted a systematic review and asked the question 'Can interventions that target yellow flags achieve better outcomes?'[7] In general, their findings suggested that if a patient was identified as having yellow flags and underwent a targeted psychological intervention, the outcomes were positive.[7] However, there is no firm consensus on how patients should be assessed for yellow flags and which flags should indicate the need for which intervention. We therefore include the section on yellow flags with the intention of making readers aware of their presence in the literature and in the clinical area of pain management, with the caveat that this strategy requires much further validation.

THE CASES

Two of the cases that follow look at using red flags in the diagnostic process. The final case, albeit an uncommon condition, gives an introduction to thinking about yellow flags when consulting.

An 82-year-old man presents with a painful, swollen, hot joint in the forefinger of his right hand. A summary of what is happening in this case in the *diagnostic initiation phase* is:

The patient is complaining of a hot, swollen joint, which should act as a pattern recognition trigger that causes you to form an initial differential diagnosis.

1 You examine the patient's hands. Describe the features shown in Figures 7.1 and 7.2.

These are the hands of an elderly man. The skin and nails are in generally good condition, although there is some dirt under the fingernails. There are a few scattered solar lentigos. There are hairs on the dorsal aspect of the hands and some prominent veins bilaterally. The patient has a swollen proximal interphalangeal joint of the index finger of the right hand. The skin over the swelling is erythematous and shiny.

Next, you refine your diagnosis by seeking to confirm the presence or absence of red flags. Consider the most common cause of this problem and then consider serious diagnoses that must be ruled out.

Your initial differential diagnosis should have included gout, pseudogout, septic arthritis and acute exacerbation of osteoarthritis.

2 What is your differential diagnosis of a hot swollen joint, and what is this most likely to be in this case?

The differential diagnosis includes gout, pseudogout, septic arthritis and an acute exacerbation of osteoarthritis. In the UK, gout is the most common inflammatory arthritis (affecting 2.5% of adults).[2]

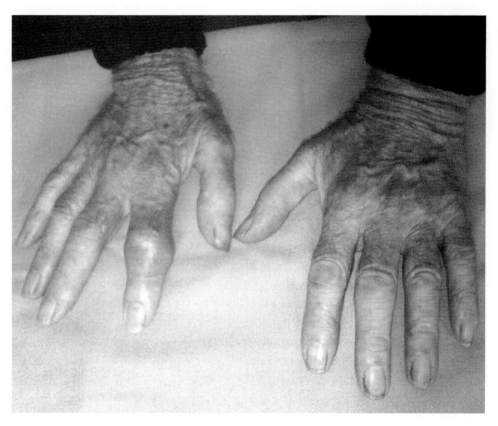

Fig. 7.1 The hands of a patient with a painful index finger.

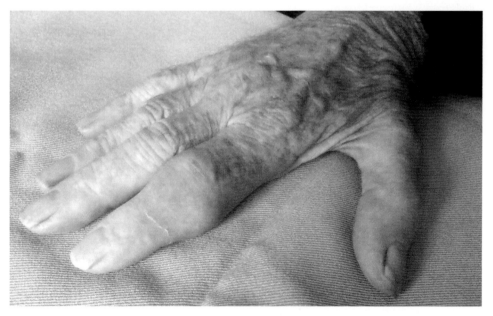

Fig. 7.2 Close-up of the patient's right hand.

3 Which red flag symptoms would you ask about in order to rule out septic arthritis?

The absence of several red flags will help rule out septic arthritis. Septic arthritis is more likely in the presence of fever, night sweats, rigors, coexistent rheumatoid arthritis, immunosuppression, joint prosthesis, intravenous drug use, structural deformity and recent bacterial infection. Also note that the proximal interphalangeal joint of the index finger is an unusual joint in which to develop septic arthritis.

The patient tells you that the onset of pain was rapid and that it was maximal in less than 24 hours. He reports no history of fever and is not systemically unwell (which you confirm by finding a normal pulse rate, blood pressure and temperature). He also tells you he has had similar episodes in the past, treated effectively by his GP with non-steroidal anti-inflammatory drugs (NSAIDs).

4 How does this help to narrow your differential diagnosis?

The nature of the pain helps you to decide whether it fits more with a diagnosis of gout or of septic arthritis. Septic arthritis tends to have a more insidious onset, whereas the pain in gout tends to come on more suddenly. In acute gout, crystals that have built up in cartilage over time spill out into the joint space, causing synovial irritation and inflammation

The patient volunteers that he thinks this is a flare of his osteoarthritis.

5 What factors would you ask about or look for that would help confirm that this is not osteoarthritis?

Several questions can be asked to help consider a possible diagnosis of osteoarthritis:

- Is there a history of trauma?
- Have they noticed any other joint swelling? (Look for Heberden's and Bouchard's nodes.)
- Have they had pain, swelling and stiffness at the base of the thumb?
- If they have hip pain, do they have any factors that predispose to hip osteoarthritis (previous Perthe's disease, leg length discrepancy, previous hip trauma)?

You suspect this is a case of gout and examine the patient further.

6 Where else might you expect to find evidence of gout?

The typical places to find gout include the first metatarsophalangeal joint (where the term *podagra* is sometimes used), tarsal and subtalar joints and larger joints such as the ankle, knee and wrist. Podagra is shown in **Figure 7.3**.

The patient was successfully treated with a short course of NSAIDs and concomitant omeprazole for gastroprotection. Remember that patients with gout have an increased risk of cardiovascular disease so it is pertinent to screen patients presenting with gout for cardiovascular risk factors.[9]

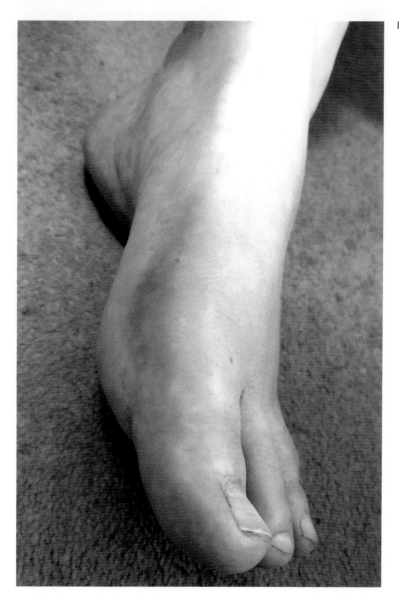

Fig. 7.3 Podagra.

A patient suffered a cerebral haemorrhage 16 years ago. He has a hemiparesis that makes walking difficult. His hands are shown in **Figure 7.4**.

Fig. 7.4A The patient's hands.

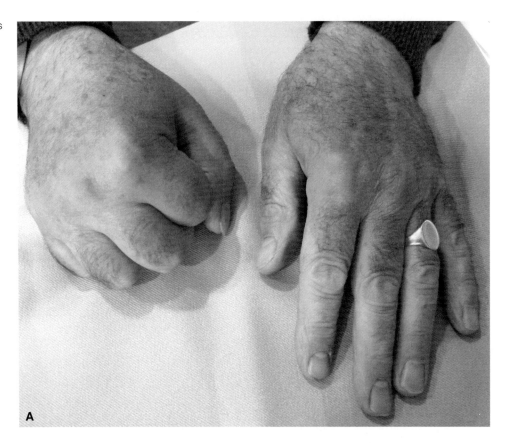

A

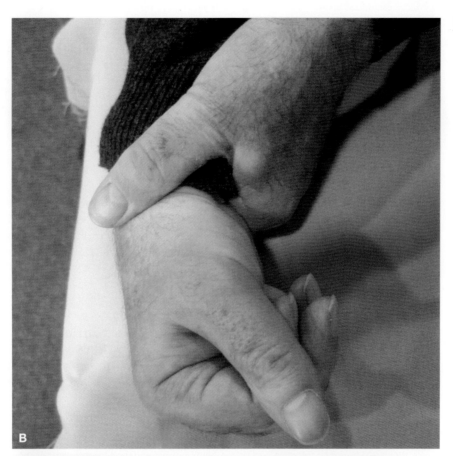

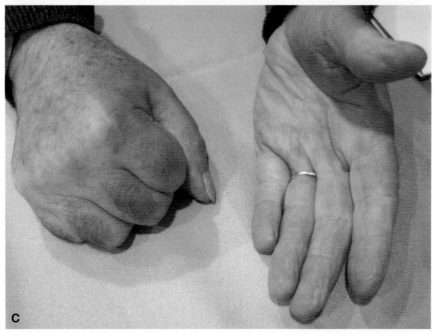

1 What features are notable in this patient's hands?

These are the hands of an elderly man. His nails are in good condition and he wears a ring on the ring finger of his left hand. The patient's right hand is slightly oedematous and there is less hair on it than on the left hand. The right hand is clenched in a fist. From the photo series, you can see that his right hand remains in this position whereas he is able to move his left hand.

2 Where was the likely location of the stroke?

Given that the stroke has affected the patient's right upper limb, the location of the stroke is likely to be the area of the brain supplied by the left middle cerebral artery.

3 If a patient is presenting with an acute stroke, time is of the essence as prompt treatment can save neurons. Which red flag features would you be looking for connected with the diagnosis of stroke?

Red flags for stroke are the following:

- There is a sudden onset of symptoms.
- 'Face, arm, speech, time' (FAST) screening is often used outside hospital (F = facial droop, A = arm weakness, S = speech difficulties, T = time to call 999).
- In hospital, current NICE guidelines advise using a validated screening tool such as the ROSIER (Recognition of Stroke in the Emergency Room) tool to screen for the red flags that, if present, point towards possible stroke. In the ROSIER tool, these features are asymmetrical facial, arm and leg weakness, speech disturbance and visual field defects.

4 What should you exclude in patients who have experienced sudden-onset neurological symptoms?

Assessment of a patient's risk of a certain problem can be achieved by a variety of means and is usually a combined approach. One method is to ask about patient characteristics that act to increase the risk of a given condition (searching for risk factors in the history). Another is to use clinical prediction rules (see Chapter 3) or to look for specific clinical signs on examination (see Chapter 5).

You should seek to exclude hypoglycaemia in patients experiencing sudden-onset neurological symptoms.

5 What risk factors for both ischaemic and haemorrhagic stroke would you ask about when taking a history from this patient?

Risk factors for ischaemic stroke are smoking, hypertension, hypercholesterolaemia, diabetes mellitus, obesity, previous history of ischaemic cardiovascular disease (e.g. myocardial infarction, ischaemic limb), cardiac disease such as atrial fibrillation, cardiomyopathy, valve disease, positive family history (and use of the combined oral contraceptive pill).

Risk factors for haemorrhagic stroke are trauma, hypertension, use of anticoagulants, disorders of coagulation and platelet abnormalities, intracerebral neoplasia, positive family history and arteriovenous malformations (such as those found in hereditary haemorrhagic telangiectasia).

6 What other diagnoses may account for this presentation (a right-sided upper limb paralysis)?

A left hemisphere space-occupying lesion may present with a right-sided upper limb paralysis.

A 35-year-old woman who works in an office sustained a minor crush injury to her left forearm. A fracture was ruled out by X-ray shortly after the injury.

Over the last 6 months she has worn her left arm in a home-made sling with an elastic wrist support and taken paracetamol as required for pain. She has been unable to work during that time and complains of persistent pain and paraesthesiae in the affected hand. She enjoys running and going to the gym but has recently been avoiding these activities. She is a single parent to two children and has been relying on her mother, who lives nearby, for support with childcare. She is worried that she is 'not getting better quickly enough'.

Her GP has ruled out other causes for her pain, and a diagnosis of complex regional pain syndrome (CRPS) has been made. When considering such a diagnosis, clinicians can refer to the clinical diagnostic criteria produced by the International Association for the Study of Pain.[10]

COMPLEX REGIONAL PAIN SYNDROME

This is an uncommon diagnosis and one of exclusion (see Chapter 3). It is a syndrome in which there is disproportionate (in terms of intensity or duration) distal limb pain and dysregulation of the microvacsculature that leads to oedema, changes in colour or problems with sweating.[11] When a specific nerve injury is identified, it is referred to as CRPS type II, and where there is no specific nerve injury, it is referred to as CRPS type I. Signs and symptoms to look for are shown in *Table 7.1*.[10] Studies have shown that it is more frequently seen in female patients and after upper limb injuries.[10]

The patient often experiences morbidity in the form of severe limitation of their activities of daily living. This can impact on their psychological well-being. At 12 months, 25% of patients still fit the criteria for the diagnosis of CRPS.[12] A combined multidisciplinary approach to CRPS that includes medical, physical, occupational and psychological therapy is usually applied.[10]

Table 7.1 Signs and symptoms of CRPS

Symptoms	Signs
Hyperalgesia	Changes to skin colour
Allodynia	Changes to skin temperature
Reduced strength	Changes to sweating
	Oedema
	Tremors
	Dystonia
	Altered proprioception in affected limb

1 The patient's hands are shown in Figures 7.5 and 7.6. What features can you identify that would be consistent with the diagnosis of CRPS?

Fig. 7.5 Dorsal aspect of the patient's hands.

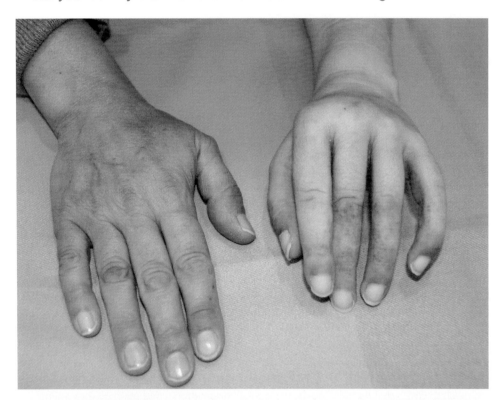

Fig. 7.6 Palmar aspect of the patient's hands.

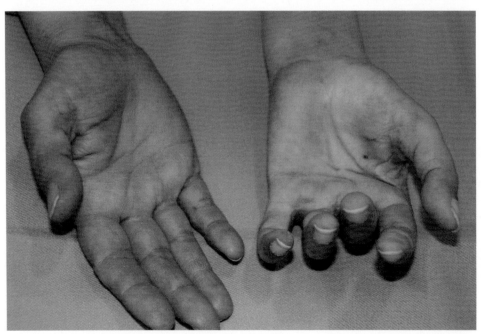

These are the hands of a young woman. The right hand looks healthy and the nails are shiny and in good condition. At the left wrist, there is evidence of mild oedema, and the impression left by the elastic wrist support can be seen. There is also wasting of the muscles in the left forearm. The skin underneath where the elastic support has been is notably lighter in colour, especially when compared with the other hand. The nails of the left hand are pale and dull. The palmar aspect of the left hand shows muscle wasting of the thenar eminence and loss of colour to the skin where the sling has rested. There is some palmar erythema, possibly due to micro-vascular changes. In both figures, the affected left hand adopts a claw-like posture.

2 Given the diagnosis of CRPS, what sorts of issue might you explore that might indicate psychological yellow flags?

Think about the three categories of psychological yellow flags (beliefs and judgements, emotional responses, pain behaviour). You might ask about:

- Beliefs and judgements: beliefs about the pain (such as fear, belief that all pain indicates injury or that pain is usually uncontrollable) and beliefs about recovery that are unhelpful (such as a belief that recovery is not possible or unlikely).[7]
- Emotional responses: whether the patient suffers from anxiety or has a tendency to catastrophise, history of depression and level of distress regarding their diagnosis.[7]
- Pain behaviour: such as the avoidance of activity due to pain.[7] In the case here, there is a history of the patient avoiding physical activity.

3 What is the cause of the forearm muscle wasting, and how might this affect this patient's recovery?

The cause of the left forearm muscle wasting is disuse atrophy.

The patient was initially referred for physiotherapy, which helped her build the strength in her forearm. This enabled her to return to work without the sling but she continued to have problems with pain. She attended a specialist pain clinic and was referred for pain-focused cognitive behavioural therapy.

SUMMARY

- This chapter details how clinicians search for red flags as markers of serious pathology to help them make sure they do not overlook a 'Do not miss' diagnosis.
- In addition, the concept of yellow flags (psychosocial factors that are associated with chronicity of symptoms and long-term disability) is introduced.
- Red flags are highlighted in two cases and yellow flags are explored in the final case.

REFERENCES

1 Heneghan C, Glasziou P, Thompson M, *et al.* Diagnostic strategies used in primary care. *BMJ* 2009;**338**:b946.
2 Adams E, Goyder C, Heneghan C, Brand L, Aijawi R. Clinical reasoning of junior doctors in emergency medicine: a grounded theory study. *Emerg Med J* 2017;**34**:70–5.
3 Murtagh J. Diagnostic modelling in general practice. *Aust Med Stud J* 2011;**2**:46–7.
4. Croskerry P, Singhal G, Mamede S. Cognitive debiasing 1: origins of bias and theory of debiasing. *BMJ Qual Saf* 2013;**22**(Suppl 2):ii58–64.
5 Goyder CR, Jones CHD, Heneghan CJ, Thompson MJ. Missed opportunities for diagnosis: lessons learned from diagnostic errors in primary care. *Br J Gen Pract* 2015;**65**:e838–44.
6 Samanta J, Kendall J, Samanta A. Chronic low back pain. *BMJ* 2003;**326**:535.
7 Nicholas MK, Linton SJ, Watson PJ, Main CJ, "Decade of the Flags" Working Group. Early identification and management of psychological risk factors ("yellow flags") in patients with low back pain: a reappraisal. *Phys Ther* 2011;**91**:737–53.
8 Krismer M, van Tulder M. Low back pain (non-specific). *Best Pract Res Clin Rheumatol* 2007;**21**:77–91.
9 Singh JA. When gout goes to the heart: does gout equal a cardiovascular disease risk factor? *Ann Rheum Dis* 2015;**74**:631.
10 Bruehl S. Complex regional pain syndrome. *BMJ* 2015;351.
11 Oaklander AL, Horowitz SH. The complex regional pain syndrome. *Handb Clin Neurol* 2015;**131**: 481–503.
12 Birklein F, Dimova V. Complex regional pain syndrome-up-to-date. *Pain Rep* 2017;**2**:e624.

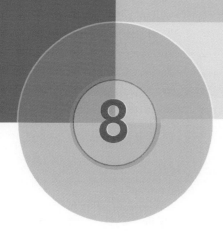

Restricted rule-outs

8

INTRODUCTION

The restricted rule-out strategy (Murtagh's process) is focused on the need to exclude a limited number of serious diagnoses.[1] It is synonymous with the 'rule out worst case scenario' (ROWS) strategy that has been identified as being employed in emergency medicine.[2] It is an example of a strategy that involves 'cognitive forcing' (see Chapter 3) and is almost uniformly relied on by clinicians in high-risk clinical environments such as emergency medicine and out of hours services.[2,3]

In the high-risk context, the focus of the differential diagnosis is a list of serious ('must rule out') conditions. Several strategies are often combined in this approach.[1] For example, knowing the likelihood of diagnoses (probabilistic reasoning) is an important factor in generating the 'rule-out list', and the use of red flags in the history and examination further assist the identification of serious conditions. It is also important to know what the most common cause of a presenting symptom is likely to be in any given clinical context.[4,5] Additionally, the clinician needs to be confident in what can be 'ruled out' based on the information gathered.

The restricted rule-out strategy uses the 'availability heuristic' – a rule of thumb that clinicians develop which involves knowing the most significant 'must rule out' diagnoses for a given presentation.[2] For example, subarachnoid haemorrhage would be included in the list of significant rule-outs for a patient with a severe headache.

By methodically ruling out the serious and being inherently biased towards looking for these serious diagnoses, this diagnostic strategy can help to reduce clinical errors and promote patient safety.[2,4] Unfortunately, on occasion, a serious illness may be ruled out when in fact it is present because the features used to rule it out have yet to develop in the patient.[1] Therefore, safety netting is key.

'SAFE' SAFETY NETTING

Proficiency in safety netting is a key skill in areas such as general practice and emergency medicine. It involves a discussion with the patient, sometimes with the addition of written information, and should include:[6]

- An acknowledgement of the existence of diagnostic uncertainty.
- What can be expected during the time course of the condition.
- Which new or evolving symptoms should prompt the patient to seek further help.
- How the patient should seek further help and in what timescale.

This discussion should be documented in the patient notes.

The cases that follow illustrate the process of developing a 'must rule out' differential diagnosis.

You are asked to see a 77-year-old man in a residential care home. His daughter has expressed her concerns to the manager that her father has a large 'bruise' on his hand.

You have a brief summary of his clinical history from the notes, including:

- A move to the care home during the last 3 months from living independently at home.
- Previous myocardial infarction 5 years ago with a stent fitted.
- Metallic heart valve fitted – the patient takes warfarin.
- Mild cognitive impairment.
- Benign prostatic hypertrophy.
- Mild osteoarthritis.

First, let us recap on definitions. The term *purpura* refers to the haemorrhage of small blood vessels in the skin or mucous membranes and can be subcategorised into petechiae (small pin-point macules), ecchymoses (larger bruises), palpable purpura (associated with vasculitis) and pigmented purpura.[7]

As discussed previously, while taking a history, we are often simultaneously gaining visual clues from the patient. You continue to talk to the patient while observing his hands.

1 How would you describe these lesions (Figures 8.1 and 8.2)?

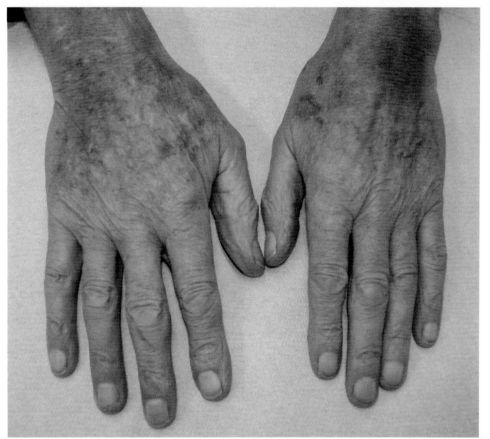

Fig. 8.1 The patient's hands.

Fig. 8.2 Close-up of the dorsal aspect of the patient's left hand.

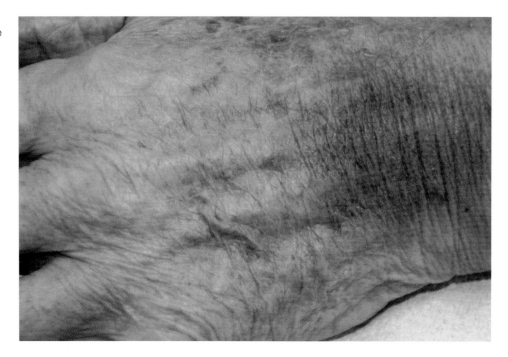

The patient has two flat lesions on the left hand consistent with ecchymoses. One is coin shaped and red in colour, the other is larger and has a purple centre with a yellow–brown border.

You ask the patient about the bruises but he cannot remember how they came about. The care home does not report any falls. He has been otherwise well and has not seen a doctor for some months.

Next consider what the differential diagnosis might be for a patient presenting with ecchymoses. The differential for bruising is wide, but in the first part of this case we are employing the restricted rule-out strategy and therefore considering ruling out serious pathology.

2 If you are employing a restricted rule-out strategy here, which serious conditions that can present with bruising need to be ruled out given the clinical context?

These include:

- An international normalised ratio (INR) in excess of the therapeutic range.
- Haematological malignancy (e.g. leukaemia).
- Disorder of the clotting cascade other than warfarinisation (probably acquired, given the age of the patient here) – note that this could be due to a problem with the elements of the clotting cascade themselves or the liver, which synthesises them.
- Thrombocytopenia (which has multiple causes such as drugs, idiopathic thrombotic thrombocytopenia and haematological malignancy).
- Non-accidental injury (NAI).

Note that if this patient was taking a direct acting oral anticoagulant consider renal dysfunction, which can cause impaired clearance of certain anticoagulant drugs such as apixaban.[8]

3 With these conditions in mind, what questions would you want to ask to establish whether there is a problem with the coagulation cascade or with platelets?

- Ask questions about mucocutaneous bleeding such as 'Have you had any nosebleeds recently?' and 'Have you noticed bleeding when you brush your teeth?' Note that, in this case, the patient has cognitive impairment so the history may need to come from his relatives and carers in the care home. Has any rash been noticed? (Here we are thinking about a petechial rash.) Mucocutaneous bleeding and petechiae point towards a platelet problem. Remember that petechiae have a number of other serious causes that need to be ruled out should you encounter them.
- Ask about bleeding from other sites, such as rectal bleeding.
- Quantify any such bleeding.

4 What features should you ask about in the history to help you rule out haematological malignancy?

The following features may point towards a potential underlying haematological malignancy:

- Weight loss.
- Recurrent infections.
- Night sweats.
- Fever.
- Lymphadenopathy.
- Bone pain.
- Symptoms of anaemia (e.g. breathlessness, fatigue).

The drug history is important in relation to clotting and platelet problems. You ask for the medication sheet for the patient, which is as follows:

- Simvastatin.
- Amlodipine.
- Warfarin.
- Paracetamol PRN ('as required').
- Tamsulosin.
- Ibuprofen PRN for osteoarthritis.

The immediate concern, given the bruising, is the warfarin therapy. Is the correct warfarin dosage regime being communicated to and followed by the care home? Paracetamol is being prescribed on an 'as required' basis; has the patient recently increased his paracetamol consumption, which might elevate the INR?[9] The ibuprofen may also be contributing (see below).

5 What factors may interfere with a patient's warfarin control?

Warfarin is primarily metabolised via the cytochrome P450 system in the liver. Enzyme-inhibiting drugs (e.g. antibiotics such as metronidazole and erythromycin, anticonvulsants such as sodium valproate, allopurinol and also paracetamol) may cause a patient's INR to increase. Enzyme-inducing drugs (e.g. sulphonylureas, carbamazepine, phenytoin) may cause a patient's INR to decrease. Alcohol in the context of binge drinking can act as an enzyme inhibitor, and in the context of chronic drinking acts as an enzyme inducer.

Always check whether the patient is taking their medication, and that they or their carers know how much should be taken and what monitoring regime is in place for their INR. Note that selective serotonin reuptake inhibitors, which are commonly prescribed antidepressants, can increase the risk of bleeding when co-prescribed with warfarin.[10] As part of the drug history, remember to ask if the patient is taking any herbal remedies that might interact with warfarin, such as St John's wort or ginko biloba.

This patient on warfarin has been co-prescribed ibuprofen.

6 For what reasons is the co-prescription of a non-steroidal anti-inflammatory drug with warfarin a significant concern?

Non-steroidal anti-inflammatory drugs inhibit the production of mucus in the stomach via inhibition of prostaglandin synthesis. This leads to an increased tendency to gastric bleeding. They also interfere with the synthesis of thromboxane A2, which affects platelet aggregation and can increase the risk of bleeding via this mechanism.

It is beyond the remit of this book to discuss the diagnosis of NAI. However, in this case, NAI forms part of the differential diagnosis of serious 'must rule outs'. It is useful therefore to think about how the pattern of bruising may point towards the possibility of NAI.[11] In general, bruising on the face and neck, forearms, back and chest, and lumbar and gluteal areas is more suggestive of elder abuse.[11] It is not reliable to try to age a bruise by looking at its colour.[11] Also think about how you would document, report and escalate your findings within the clinical context in which you are working should you suspect NAI.

In the above case, there are no features to suggest NAI. On questioning the patient and his carers, no symptoms suggestive of haematological malignancy are reported. There are no reports of bleeding from elsewhere.

You examine the patient for other injuries and bruising (in particular remembering to consider the possibility of associated intracranial bleeding [e.g. a chronic subdural haemorrhage]).

There are no other bruises or injuries and the patient appears very well in himself. Heart rate, respiratory rate and blood pressure are normal.

A focused history and examination has helped you start to rule out the serious conditions mentioned above.

7 What investigations would you now request?

It would be sensible to request a full blood count and clotting profile (including INR), urea and electrolytes.

These investigations are all normal. The patient's INR is 3.2.

8 What conclusions do you make regarding the patient's lesions?

The patient has an INR in the target range but by virtue of the fact that he is taking an anti-coagulant, he is more prone to easy bruising. Hence the lesions on the left hand and wrist likely represent purpura associated with warfarin therapy (more likely to occur in patients with advancing years due to skin fragility).

A NOTE ABOUT SENILE PURPURA

This is a condition of bruising secondary to minor trauma that occurs in elderly individuals due to collagen changes in the skin, which leads to extravasation of blood into the dermis.[12] The changes are a result of chronic sun exposure and ageing and hence these lesions are more common in sun-exposed areas such as the backs of the hands.[12] They are dark purple in appearance and do not undergo the normal colour changes of other bruises (compare this with the lesion in this patient, which shows yellowing at the peripheries).

Case 8.2

An 80-year-old man presents to his GP with a skin lesion on the dorsum of his hand. He says it has been there some months and is mildly itchy.

To illustrate the restricted rule-out strategy, we need to form a list of differential diagnoses. The lesion may be malignant, benign with malignant potential or benign.

1 What types of lesion would be on your differential diagnosis list in each category (malignant, benign with malignant potential and benign)?

Table 8.1 shows the differential diagnoses.

Table 8.1 Categorisation of skin lesions

Malignant	Benign with malignant potential	Benign
Melanoma	Solar (actinic) keratosis	Viral wart
Squamous cell carcinoma	Bowen's disease (although more common on the legs, especially in women)	Seborrhoeic keratosis
Basal cell carcinoma (less likely on the hand)	Keratoacanthoma	Pyogenic granuloma
Cutaneous metastases	Lentigo maligna (although this typically occurs on the face)	Cutaneous neurofibroma
Cutaneous lymphoma	Atypical moles	Keloid scar
		Angioma

You take a short history from the patient. He says he often scratches the top off the lesion but it comes back. He says he cannot remember exactly how long it has been there but he thinks for several months. He is worried about skin cancer as his friend was recently diagnosed with a skin cancer on his face.

2 What questions might you ask that determine whether the patient has risk factors for skin cancer?

- Have you ever lived or worked in a hot country?
- What sort of skin have you got – do you tan easily or burn? (Think about the Fitzpatrick skin types: https://www.dermnetnz.org/topics/skin-phototype/.)
- Did or do you have a job outdoors?
- Have you ever been badly sunburnt, particularly as a child?
- Have you ever used sunbeds?
- Has anyone in your family suffered from a skin cancer?
- Past medical history is relevant. Has the patient previously had a skin cancer? Note that squamous cell carcinoma (SCC) is more common in people with psoriasis, and skin tumours are more common in patients taking immunosuppressant drugs or suffering from an immunosuppressive condition such as chronic lymphocytic leukaemia.

3 What risk factors for skin cancer might you discern on observation of the patient?

- Fair skin.
- Red hair.
- Freckling.
- Multiple melanocytic naevi.

4 You examine the patient's hands. What observations can you make from Figure 8.3?

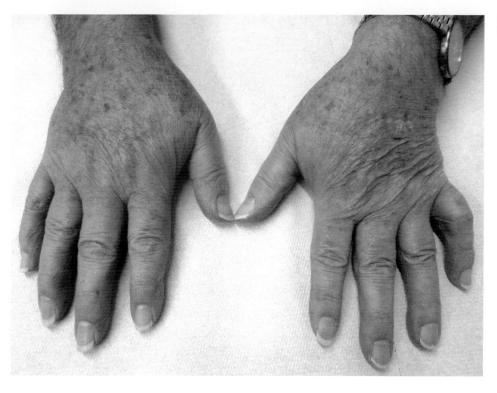

Fig. 8.3 The patient's hands.

These are the hands of an elderly man. The nails look like they are in good condition. He has multiple solar lentigines over both hands and a scaly lesion on the dorsum of the left hand. He appears to have a flexion deformity of the proximal interphalangeal joint of the little finger of the left hand.

5 Looking at Figure 8.4, describe the lesion on the dorsum of the left hand.

Fig. 8.4 The lesion on the dorsum of the left hand.

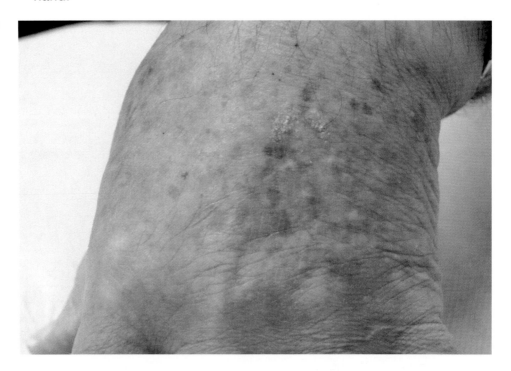

There is a keratotic, scaly papule on the dorsum of the left hand.

6 What tools can help you identify skin cancers?

These include:

- The 'ABCDE rule' for looking at suspicious melanocytic lesions (A = asymmetry, B = irregular border, C = variation in colour, D = diameter >7 mm, E = evolving lesion) helps to identify lesions with alarm features.
- Knowledge of the typical clinical features of different skin cancers (e.g. basal cell carcinomas often look pearly with a smooth surface and visible blood vessels).
- Dermoscopy (if you are fully trained in this).
- Photography including dermoscopic photographs sent for review by a dermatologist via an email advice line.
- Referral to a dermatology 'suspected skin tumour' clinic.
- Biopsy and specimen sent for histopathological diagnosis.

Given its appearance, the lesion is unlikely to be a melanoma (although always remember that amelanocytic melanoma is a subtype of melanoma).

You ask questions about previous sun exposure. The patient tells you he had an office job when younger but spent a lot of holidays abroad and did not really use sun cream.

7 What questions would you ask specifically about the lesion?

Ask about itching, bleeding and whether the lesion has changed and/or increased in size.

We know that it is mildly itchy (see above). He reports that the lesion has not grown over the past 6–8 weeks.

8 Can you make a diagnosis of the lesion on the left hand?

Given the appearance of the lesion, the history of sun exposure with multiple solar lentigines and the absence of red flags for skin malignancy (such as the presence of an evolving lesion – bleeding, growing, ulcerating – and features consistent with the ABCDE rule), a clinical diagnosis of a solar (actinic) keratosis could be made. Remember to palpate the skin in dermatological examinations. Solar keratoses often feel rough like sandpaper and can often be felt before they can be seen.[13]

Another useful clinical pointer is a lack of induration, which is reassuring. SCCs are often tender or painful and indurated whereas solar keratoses are usually not.

In addition, solar keratoses are extremely common in white individuals, especially those of advanced age who often had a lot of sun exposure prior to the development of sun cream and sun safety advice. These lesions appear in sun-exposed sites such as the dorsum of the hand, adding credence to the diagnosis here.

You explain that solar keratoses can be treated with cryotherapy, creams such as 5-fluorouracil, photodynamic therapy and surgery. You also advise the patient that he might get further solar keratoses but from now on he should try to practise sun safety. There are useful patient resources on this topic that can be given to the patient, such as sun safety leaflets produced by the British Association of Dermatologists.

Remember that solar keratoses do not all necessarily need to be treated, especially when mild and in elderly patients.

In this case, the lesion was treated successfully with cryotherapy.

9 How might you provide a safety net for the patient?

Refer to the guidance at the beginning of the chapter on safe safety netting. Provision of written information can be really helpful here. For example, the British Association of Dermatologists has online patient information leaflets that can be downloaded and printed. You should advise the patient about the following:

- Diagnostic uncertainty: explain that all the current signs and symptoms point towards this lesion being a solar keratosis.
- Time course: explain that a solar keratosis can usually be successfully treated but if left untreated a small proportion of cases can progress to a skin cancer (SCC). This is usually clinically obvious, for example with the development of a nodule.
- When should the patient seek further help: advise that it is good to check the skin every couple of months for new lesions or changes to the skin. If the patient notices any changes, he should seek advice. The features that should prompt the patient to seek further advice from the GP should be explained (e.g. new, growing, itching, bleeding lesions and the ABCDE features for melanocytic lesions).
- Where to seek help: explain that the patient should initially return to his GP if he is concerned about a skin lesion.

SUMMARY

- This chapter focuses on the restricted rule-out or 'rule out worst case scenario' strategy and emphasises the key skill of safety netting at the end of a consultation.
- The first case applies the restricted rule-out strategy and the second case explores benign and malignant skin lesions.

REFERENCES

1   Thompson MJ, Harnden A, Mar CD. Excluding serious illness in feverish children in primary care: restricted rule-out method for diagnosis. *BMJ* 2009;**338**:b1187.
2   Croskerry P. Achieving quality in clinical decision making: cognitive strategies and detection of bias. *Acad Emerg Med* 2002;**9**:1184–204.
3   Balla J, Heneghan C, Thompson M, Balla M. Clinical decision making in a high-risk primary care environment: a qualitative study in the UK. *BMJ Open* 2012;**2**:e000414.
4   Heneghan C, Glasziou P, Thompson M, *et al.* Diagnostic strategies used in primary care. *BMJ* 2009;**338**:b946.
5   Goyder CR, Jones CHD, Heneghan CJ, Thompson MJ. Missed opportunities for diagnosis: lessons learned from diagnostic errors in primary care. *Br J Gen Pract* 2015;**65**:e838–44.
6   Almond S, Mant D, Thompson M. Diagnostic safety-netting. *Br J Gen Pract* 2009;**59**:872–4.
7   Yi Zhen Chiang N, Verbov J. *Dermatology: A Handbook for Medical Students and Junior Doctors.* London: British Association of Dermatologists; 2014.
8   National Institute of Health and Care Excellence. *Bruising. Clinical Knowledge Summary.* 2016. Available from https://cks.nice.org.uk/bruising.
9   Mahe I, Bertrand N, Drouet L, *et al.* Interaction between paracetamol and warfarin in patients: a double-blind, placebo-controlled, randomized study. *Haematologica* 2006;**91**:1621.
10 Sansone RA, Sansone LA. Warfarin and antidepressants: happiness without hemorrhaging. *Psychiatry (Edgmont)* 2009;**6**:24–9.
11 Lachs MS, Pillemer KA. Elder abuse. *New Engl J Med* 2015;**373**:1947–56.
12 Hafsi W, Badri T. Actinic purpura. Updated 2018 Dec 5. Available from https://www.ncbi.nlm.nih.gov/books/NBK448130/.
13 Chetty P, Choi F, Mitchell T. Primary care review of actinic keratosis and its therapeutic options: a global perspective. *Dermatol Ther (Heidelb)* 2015;**5**:19–35.

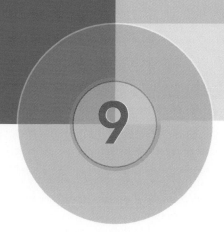

Probabilistic reasoning

INTRODUCTION

In its pure form, probabilistic reasoning is a form of analytic rather than intuitive reasoning and is based on logic, inference and probability.[1] In an ideal mathematical world, we would calculate the probabilities of the conditions in our differential diagnosis, compare them and select the most probable.[2] This is not practical in clinical practice, and as Black *et al.* eloquently put it, 'The bottom line is that clinicians can provide the highest quality care by maximising their use of various decision-making tools and by integrating information derived from various quantitative approaches with their own clinical judgement.'[3] Heneghan *et al.* reported in their study of diagnostic strategies used by GPs that probabilistic reasoning was one of five strategies employed in the refinement stage of diagnosis.[4] However, it is a strategy that is rarely applied consciously, in contrast to (for example) running through a checklist of red flags when faced with a patient with a particular presenting complaint.

USING PROBABILITIES IN CLINICAL REASONING

Clinicians use probabilistic reasoning at two stages in the diagnostic process. First, we consider the *likelihood* that a patient has a given condition when we refine our differential diagnosis (this is usually done intuitively and not by calculating actual probabilities).[5] Second, we use it to consider whether to request further investigations.[5]

In terms of refining the differential diagnosis, the clinician first needs to know or have an idea of the 'pretest probability' that a patient has a condition based on the information they have gleaned from the history and examination. This primarily comes through experience of patients with similar conditions and knowledge of the working context. Supporting information can be accumulated by looking for factors such as a positive family history or relevant lifestyle factors, which may increase the likelihood that a disease is present, or by using a formal clinical prediction rule (see Chapter 3). We should be particularly cautious when evaluating patients who seem to be presenting in an unusual way.

Making the decision to request a particular test requires a knowledge of how well the test might modify the probability of a condition being present (i.e. a knowledge of the sensitivity and specificity of a test).[3] One example is the use of a D-dimer test. The Cochrane Library has systematically reviewed its use for the exclusion of pulmonary embolism.[6] D-dimers (fibrin degradation products) are elevated in the presence of a deep venous thrombosis or pulmonary embolus but may also be elevated in many other conditions such as malignancy and pregnancy, as well as in patients aged more than 65 years and those who smoke.

Since the test has a high sensitivity (>95%), it can be used in conjunction with a pretest probability calculation to help rule out venous thromboembolism (VTE).[7] A negative D-dimer test has a high negative predictive value, so if a patient has a low pretest probability of VTE as calculated by their Well's score (a VTE-specific clinical prediction rule – see Chapter 3), requesting a D-dimer is appropriate. A D-dimer result less than 500 μg/L in this situation would help to rule out the diagnosis of VTE.

Remember that clinicians must, however, always consider the full clinical picture. One helpful approach is for clinicians to ask themselves, 'How might this test alter my management of this patient?', rather than adopting a scatter gun approach to requesting investigations.

THINKING ABOUT A DIAGNOSTIC PROCESS THAT USES PROBABILISTIC REASONING

Llewelyn *et al.* describe 'leads', which can be seen as the first stage in probabilistic reasoning.[8] 'Leads' or 'pivots' described by Eddy and Clanton are findings that have a limited number of conditions associated with them.[2] These findings may be symptoms, signs or results of tests. They are the starting point for collecting further information to form a 'predictive combination'.

For example, if the lead is 'cough', you might collect the following – the cough is productive of green sputum and associated with a fever and lethargy, dullness to percussion of the right lung base and bronchial breathing on auscultation of the right lung base. Using the 'lead' or 'pivot' (e.g. productive cough), one can think of differential diagnoses that might fit. At this stage, the differential diagnosis can be wide and does not need to consider the probability that the condition caused the 'lead'.[2]

This differential diagnosis is then refined by considering the predictive combination (e.g. green sputum, fever, lethargy, dullness to percussion, bronchial breathing); a diagnosis is selected and then validated.[2] In the refinement stage of the diagnostic process, clinicians are again unlikely to calculate probabilities explicitly but generally compare their knowledge of the characteristics of diseases and predictive combinations with the characteristics of the patient.

Have a think about the following cases, which draw upon these ideas.

A 70-year-old woman presents with generalised marked pain and stiffness in her hands.

1 With this presenting complaint, what leads might you look for in the history and examination?

Possible leads are:

- A history of polyarthritis.
- A history of early morning stiffness (defined as stiffness lasting more than 30 minutes).
- Symmetrical symptoms.
- Signs and symptoms consistent with synovitis: pain (worse with rest and lack of movement), swelling (feels 'boggy' on palpation), stiffness, erythema and heat.

2 What differential diagnosis would you have in mind given a history consistent with synovitis?

Your differential diagnosis might include:

- Osteoarthritis (OA).
- Rheumatoid arthritis (RA).
- Viral-associated arthritis.
- Polyarticular gout.
- Connective tissue disease.

3 What factors in the history might increase the likelihood of rheumatoid arthritis?

Factors that increase the likelihood of RA are:

- A positive family history of RA.
- Female patient.
- Symmetrical distribution of the joints affected.
- Morning stiffness lasting over 30 minutes.
- A history of symptoms consistent with synovitis.
- Involvement of the feet.

It is important to consider the prevalence (proportion of cases at a given time) of the disease in the population when considering the likelihood of a diagnosis. In the UK the prevalence of RA in women has been estimated as 1.16%, and in men as 0.44%.[9]

On further questioning, the patient tells you she has had recent swelling in the small joints of both hands for the last 2 weeks with stiffness that is worse after resting, for example when she gets up in the morning and when she has been sitting watching TV.

The National Institute for Health and Care Excellence mentions three features that increase the *likelihood* that the cause of a patient's synovitis is due to RA:

- A greater number of joints affected.
- Inability to make a fist or flex the fingers.
- Positive MCP test.

Note the wording here – being able to identify each of the above in a patient should raise your clinical suspicion of RA, but the presence of these features is *not* diagnostic.

4 How do you perform the metacarpophalangeal (MCP) test?

This test involves gently squeezing the MCP joints and assessing for discomfort (**Figure 9.1**).

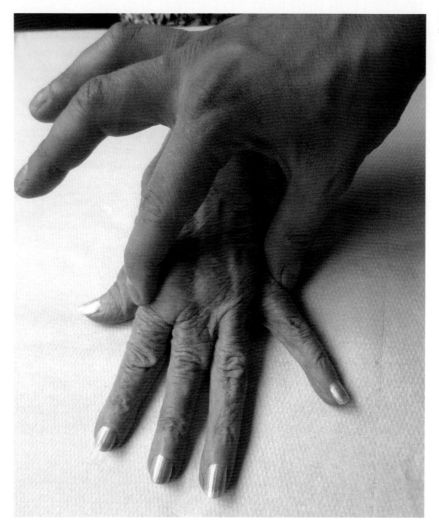

Fig. 9.1 The MCP squeeze test.

The patient in question has a positive MCP squeeze test, she has a history of symmetrical synovitis in the hands and she also mentions she has recently been feeling more fatigued. You suspect RA.

5 What blood tests would you consider to help you confirm a diagnosis of RA?

TESTING FOR RHEUMATOID FACTOR AND ANTI-CCP WHEN MAKING DIAGNOSES

It is important when requesting blood tests to consider how useful the results will be. Here we are considering the extent to which a positive test might modify the probability of a given disease being present (i.e. a knowledge of the sensitivity and specificity of a test is required). In the case of testing for rheumatoid factors, these are either IgM or IgG antibodies that are positive in 50–80% of patients with RA.[10] However, they can also occur in up to 10% of the healthy population, in patients with chronic infections and in those with autoimmune disease.[11] A positive test for rheumatoid factor therefore has a reasonably low specificity (approximately 66%).[10] This compares with a specificity of 97.9% for anti-CCP (anti-cyclic citrullinated peptide) in the diagnosis of RA.[10]

Although blood tests can be helpful, if clinical suspicion is high a GP should not delay referring a patient to a rheumatologist with a view to starting disease-modifying antirheumatic drugs. In secondary care, rheumatologists will use criteria such as the 2010 American College of Rheumatology/European League Against Rheumatism (ACR/EULAR) classification criteria for diagnosing RA.[12]

Blood tests to include here are therefore:

- C-reactive protein concentration and erythrocyte sedimentation rate.
- Rheumatoid factor.
- Anti-CCP.

THE PATIENT WITH CHRONIC RA

Long-term characteristic changes in the hands allow for pattern recognition to be used and a spot diagnosis to be made in the patient with RA. When you see a patient with such features, remember the impact of them on the patient: How are they coping with their activities of daily living? How are they coping with living with a chronic disease? How is their mood?

6 What features consistent with RA would you look for on examination of the joints in the hands and feet, and the knees?

Features consistent with RA are listed in *Table 9.1*. This patient has had RA for 18 years.

Table 9.1 Musculoskeletal features of RA (adapted from the *Oxford Handbook of Clinical Diagnosis*)[8]

Hands	Knees	Feet
Swan neck deformity	Valgus deformity	Subluxation of the metatarsal heads
Boutonnière deformity	Varus deformity	Hallux valgus
Z-thumb deformity	Baker's cysts	Clawed toes
Subluxation of the MCP joints leading to ulnar deviation		Calluses
Subluxation of the wrist joint leading to ulnar deviation		

7 Look at Figures 9.2 and 9.3. Which features of RA can you identify in this patient's hands?

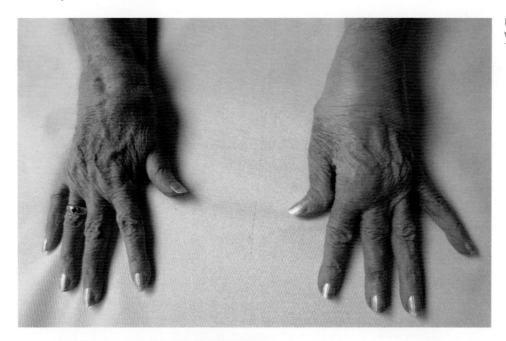

Fig. 9.2 A patient who has had RA for 18 years.

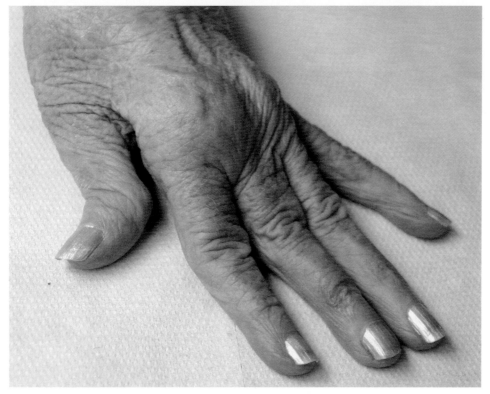

Fig. 9.3 The patient's left hand.

Identifiable features in the figures are:

- A Z-shaped thumb (with surgical scar on the left hand).
- Mild radial deviation at the wrist.
- Swelling of the left wrist.
- Left hand: volar subluxation of the MCP joints, leading to prominence of the metacarpal heads.
- Early swan neck deformity in left middle finger.
- Early ulnar deviation of the MCP joints.
- Swollen second and third MCP joints (**Figure 9.4**).
- Signs of extensor tenosynovitis at the wrist: note that this is more likely to be florid extensor tenosynovitis than synovitis at the wrist, and it could also represent chronic synovial hypertrophy.
- Wasting of the thenar eminence (**Figure 9.5**).
- Deformity at the wrist.
- Surgical scars (**Figures 9.6** and **9.7**).

Fig. 9.4A, B The patient's left wrist.

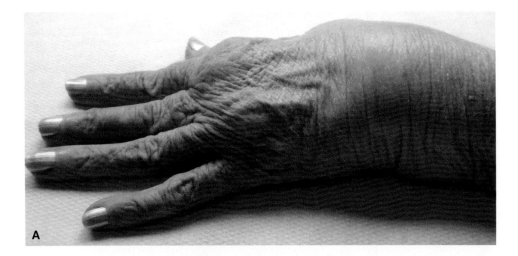

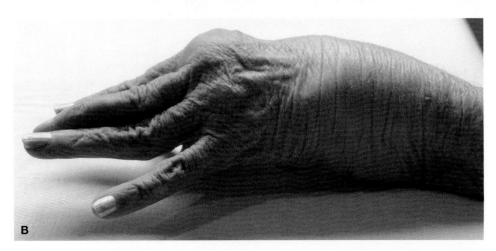

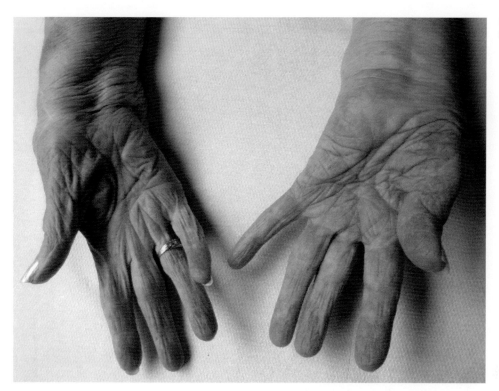

Fig. 9.5 The palmar aspect of the hands.

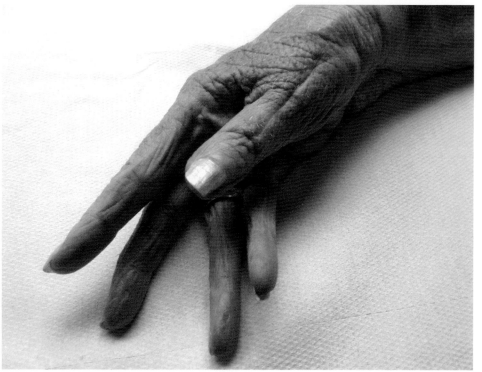

Fig. 9.6 The patient's right hand.

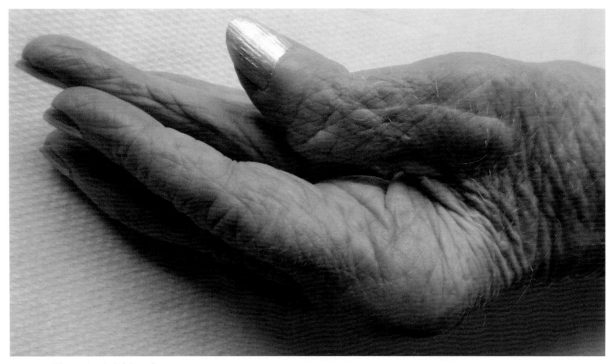

Fig. 9.7 The patient's left hand.

8 From Figures 9.4–9.7, what type of surgery do you think the patient has had?

The patient has had previous tendon surgery. Remember that carpal tunnel syndrome can be associated with RA so also look for scars at the wrist in patients with RA.

In addition, remember when examining the patient with RA to look for extra-articular manifestations and for complications of the treatments.

9 What extra-articular manifestations of RA and complications of treatment would you look for?

These are listed in *Table 9.2*.

Table 9.2 Extra-articular features and complications of RA and its treatments

Body system/location	Features
Eyes	Dry eyes as part of secondary Sjögren's syndrome
	Scleritis
	Episcleritis
	Scleromalacia perforans
	Cataracts (secondary to corticosteroids)
	Corneal deposits or retinopathy (secondary to chloroquine treatment)
Skin	Rheumatoid nodules (generally associated with seropositive disease)
	Purpura (secondary to vasculitis or corticosteroids)
	Pyoderma gangrenosum
Musculoskeletal system	Carpal tunnel syndrome
	Tendon ruptures
	Tenosynovitis
	Neck – atlantoaxial subluxation
Cardiovascular system	Increased risk of cardiovascular disease (primarily ischaemic heart disease) – look for, for example, scars from coronary artery bypass procedures
Respiratory system	Rheumatoid nodules
	Lung fibrosis (may be secondary to methotrexate treatment)
	Pleural effusions
	Caplan's syndrome (rheumatoid lung nodules + pneumoconiosis)
Central nervous system	Depression
Haematological system	Anaemia
	Increased risk of infection
	Myeloproliferative disease
	Felty's syndrome (RA + splenomegaly + neutropenia)

Note that although rheumatoid disease is often abbreviated (as we have done) to 'RA', you should always remember that it is a systemic, whole-body condition and not just an arthritis.

Case 9.2

A 70-year-old woman presents with a history of pain and stiffness in the hands over some months. She is right handed and reports her symptoms are worse on the right.

You suspect a form of arthritis.

1 Thinking about the prevalence of the different forms of arthritis, which form is most likely?

Osteoarthritis. This condition affects 70% of 70-year-olds.[13]

You ask further questions regarding the history. The patients tells you she has had pain in the hands on and off for a couple of years but recently it has become worse. Her hands are more painful towards the end of the day. She has noticed her hands are weaker and she is finding difficulty opening jars and doing the buttons on her shirt. She has tried simple analgesics, which ease but do not fully take away the pain. She finds the pain worsens with movement and rest helps it a great deal.

You ask her whether there is any family history of arthritis. She says yes, her mother suffered terribly with arthritis in her hands and knees in later life.

2 How could a question regarding family history be refined to help you further with assessing the probability that this patient has OA?

You could ask more specifically, 'Do you know what sort of arthritis your mother had? Was it rheumatoid arthritis or osteoarthritis, or another kind?'

3 What risk factors for developing OA might you ask about that, if present, would increase the probability of the patient having the condition? Hint: think about the distinction between primary and secondary OA.

Risk factors to ask about are:

- Age (there is an increasing risk of OA over the age of 60 years).
- Previous injury to the limbs (typically leg fracture), which affects the biomechanics and increases susceptibility to secondary OA.[14]
- Obesity (which increases the likelihood of secondary OA in weight-bearing joints).[14]
- A positive family history (there is increasing evidence of a genetic preponderance to OA).[14]
- An occupation involving repetitive movements (e.g. working in the clothing industry), which increases the likelihood of developing secondary OA.[15]
- A past medical history of congenital dislocation of the hip.

The further information you have gathered is helping you to put together a 'predictive combination'. This might include the following:

- In the hands, the distal interphalangeal joints are likely to be involved in OA (whereas these tend to be spared in RA).
- OA is more likely if the hips and knees are particularly affected or if only one or two joints are affected.
- In OA, the stiffness is worse with movement, relieved by rest and worse towards the end of the day.

4 What do you notice from the photograph of this patient's right hand (Figure 9.8)?

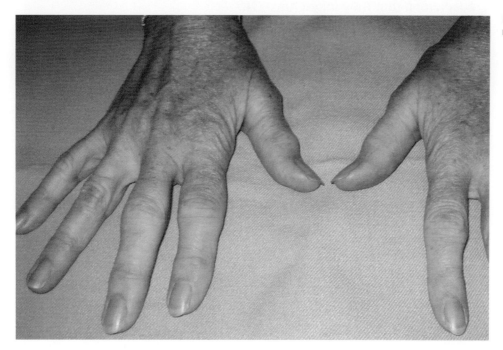

Fig. 9.8 The patient's right hand.

The second and third proximal interphalangeal joints are swollen but this represents bony swelling and is a good discriminator from RA.

HOW CAN WE DIAGNOSE OA?

EULAR has suggested that a combined approach taking into account clinical findings and presentation, risk factors elicited and radiographic features should be employed to diagnose OA.[15] It should be noted, however, that symptoms of OA may be present before changes are discernible on X-ray so clinical presentation alone is sometimes used to make a diagnosis.[15] For OA in the hands, the ACR states that the criteria for making a diagnosis are pain, aching or stiffness in the hands plus three from a list of specific joint features (such as swelling and hard tissue enlargement).[16]

OSTEOARTHRITIS OF THE BASE OF THUMB

A different patient presents with a history of pain in the radial aspect of the left thumb. He is left handed. You suspect OA of the base of the thumb (the carpometacarpal joint or, more specifically, the trapeziometacarpal joint).

5 What features of OA of the base of thumb would you seek in the history and on examination of a patient to help confirm your suspicions that they might have OA?

You should seek a history of pain and weakness of the thumb. Specifically, the pain is exacerbated by pinching or gripping actions. On examination, you might detect crepitus with tenderness at the carpometacarpal joint.[17]

Over time, 'squaring or shouldering' (a sloping prominence) develops at the base of the thumb (**Figure 9.9** of this second patient; compare the thumb bases in the two hands).[17] Here there is subluxation of the left thumb with 'squaring' of the thumb base.

Fig. 9.9 OA of the carpometacarpal joint.

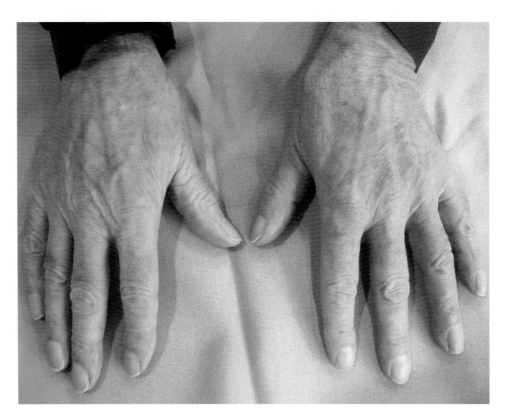

THE PATIENT WITH LONG-STANDING OSTEOARTHRITIS

As with RA, long-term characteristic changes in the hands allow for pattern recognition to be used and a spot diagnosis of specific features to be made in the patient with OA.

6 Look at this patient's hands (Figure 9.10). What features are consistent with OA? What other observations can you make?

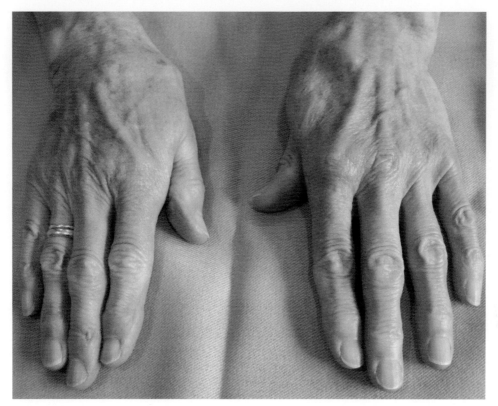

Fig. 9.10 A patient with OA.

Observations are:

- Early Heberden's and Bouchard's nodes.
- Subluxation of the thumb of the left hand.
- Bilateral squaring of the base of the thumbs.
- Muscle wasting of the dorsal interossei (most prominent in the left hand).
- Other observations: the patient wears a ring on the right hand, the skin and nails look in good condition, and there are a few scattered solar lentigos on the dorsum of the hands.

7 When you look at the palmar aspect of this patient's right hand (Figure 9.11), what else do you notice?

Fig. 9.11 The palmar aspect of the right hand.

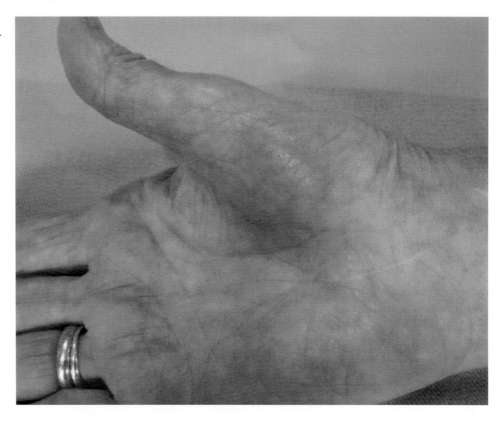

There is a scar from a carpal tunnel release procedure. Also note that there is squaring of the carpometacarpal joint.

8 Look at this next patient's hands (Figure 9.12). What features of OA are present? What other observations can you make?

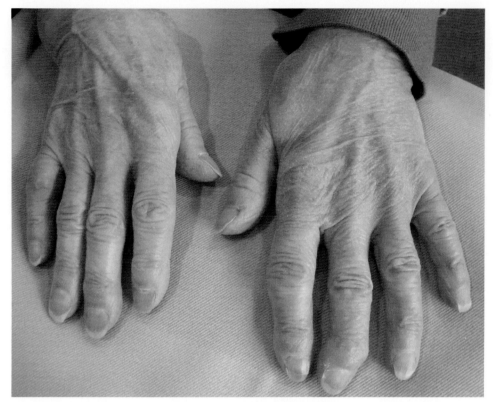

Fig. 9.12 Features of OA.

- There are Heberden's and Bouchard's nodes.
- There is rotational deformity at the distal interphalangeal joint of the middle finger on the left hand.
- There is bilateral squaring of the bases of the thumbs.
- Other observations: this is an elderly patient. The skin looks dry and thin over the dorsal aspect of the hands. The veins can easily be seen on both hands. The nails are manicured and are in good condition.

USING YOUR OBSERVATION SKILLS

Remember that OA can also affect the feet.

9 List the features that can be observed in this patient's feet
   (Figure 9.13; the features are not all necessarily related to OA).

Fig. 9.13A, B
The patient's feet.

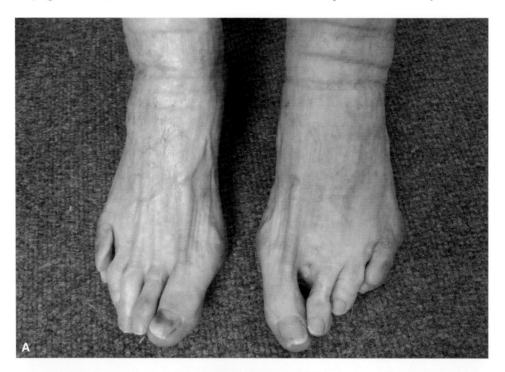

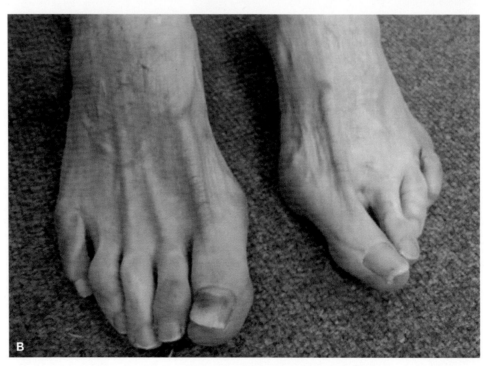

Features seen are:

- Likely *Pseudomonas* infection of the right great toenail.
- Deformity of the toe joints.
- Very mild bilateral pitting oedema: think about the possible causes for this (e.g. cardiac failure, liver disease, drugs such as calcium channel blockers).
- Bilateral hallux valgus.
- Bilateral fungal nail disease of the great toes.
- Missing toe on the left foot: think about the causes – could it be congenital or an amputation? In this patient, a scar is visible indicating amputation. This could be due to trauma or other causes such as peripheral vascular disease.

SUMMARY

- This chapter explores how we can use probabilities in clinical reasoning. For example, 'pretest probability' in the context of probabilistic reasoning is explained, along with the use of clinical prediction rules.
- The chapter describes 'leads' or 'pivots', which are findings that have a limited number of conditions associated with them.
- These ideas are applied in two rheumatological cases.

REFERENCES

1 Kassirer JP. Teaching clinical reasoning: case-based and coached. *Acad Med* 2010;**85**:1118–24.

2 Eddy DM, Clanton CH. The art of diagnosis. *New Engl J Med* 1982;**306**:1263–8.

3 Black ER, Bordley DR, Tape TG, Panzer RJ. *Diagnostic Strategies for Common Medical Problems.* Philadelphia: American College of Physicians; 1999.

4 Heneghan C, Glasziou P, Thompson M, *et al.* Diagnostic strategies used in primary care. *BMJ* 2009;**338**:b946.

5 Doust J. Using probabilistic reasoning. *BMJ* 2009;**339**:b3823.

6 Crawford F, Andras A, Welch K, Sheares K, Keeling D, Chappell FM. D-dimer test for excluding the diagnosis of pulmonary embolism. *Cochrane Database Syst Rev* 2016(8):CD010864.

7 Pulivarthi S, Gurram MK. Effectiveness of D-dimer as a screening test for venous thromboembolism: an update. *N Am J Med Sci* 2014;**6**:491–9.

8 Llewelyn H, Ang HA, Lewis K, Al-Abdulla A. *Oxford Handbook of Clinical Diagnosis.* Oxford: Oxford University Press; 2007.

9 Symmons D, Turner G, Webb R, *et al.* The prevalence of rheumatoid arthritis in the United Kingdom: new estimates for a new century. *Rheumatology* 2002;**41**:793–800.

10 Conigliaro P, Chimenti MS, Triggianese P, *et al.* Autoantibodies in inflammatory arthritis. *Autoimmun Rev* 2016;**15**:673–83.

11 Sutton B, Corper A, Bonagura V, Taussig M. The structure and origin of rheumatoid factors. *Immunol Today* 2000;**21**:177–83.

12 van der Helm-van Mil AHM, Zink A. What is rheumatoid arthritis? Considering consequences of changed classification criteria. *Ann Rheum Dis* 2017;**76**:315.

13 Kalra PA. *Essential Revision Notes for MRCP*, 3rd ed. Knutsford: Jaypee Brothers Medical Publishers.

14 Glyn-Jones S, Palmer AJR, Agricola R, *et al.* Osteoarthritis. *Lancet* 2015;**386**:376–87.

15 Leung GJ, Rainsford KD, Kean WF. Osteoarthritis of the hand I: aetiology and pathogenesis, risk factors, investigation and diagnosis. *J Pharm Pharmacol* 2014;**66**:339–46.

16 Altman R, Alarcón G, Appelrouth D, *et al.* The American College of Rheumatology criteria for the classification and reporting of osteoarthritis of the hand. *Arthritis Rheum* 1990;**33**:1601–10.

17 Swigart CR. Arthritis of the base of the thumb. *Curr Rev Musculoskelet Med* 2008;**1**:142–6.

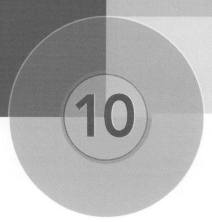

Test of time and test of treatment

10

INTRODUCTION

As discussed earlier, different strategies can be employed at different stages of the diagnostic process.[1] In the final stage, when the diagnosis is being defined, 'test of time' and 'test of treatment' strategies can be employed.

TEST OF TIME

This involves a 'watch and wait' approach and is largely employed by GPs who have the facility to review patients over varying time periods (e.g. a patient seen in the morning could be asked to return that afternoon or in 2 weeks time). Using time as a diagnostic tool is non-invasive and less costly than requesting investigations, but it should clearly never be used when the patient's presentation requires an immediate referral or treatment.[2]

The key is that, by using time and by reviewing patients on further occasions, the certainty with which the initial diagnosis has been made can be increased.[2] This occurs through analysis of whether the patient's signs and symptoms have resolved or evolved, or new features are presenting; hence we need to know the natural course of the conditions in our differential diagnosis.[2]

The test of time strategy is more often used in primary care because patients tend to present earlier in their illness and it is generally easier to arrange flexible follow-up. It can be difficult early on in a presentation to separate self-limiting from progressive illness, and hence the consideration of red flags and careful safety netting should always be employed as well. Test of time is most effective when the clinician is able to provide continuity of care.[2] It is very helpful if the same clinician reviews the patient subsequently but, for a variety of reasons, this is unfortunately not always possible hence good record keeping is essential.

TEST OF TREATMENT

This strategy is used in the end stages of making a diagnosis. Glasziou *et al.* point out that it is particularly useful when there is an atypical presentation and when there is a wide differential diagnosis.[3] We are using a 'test of treatment' when a clinical diagnosis has been made and a treatment is prescribed, such as an antifungal cream for a rash that is a suspected tinea infection. Test of treatment can be a very useful tool but beware false-positive results (e.g. due to the emollient effect of an antifungal cream or a placebo effect) and false-negative results (which can occur due to poor patient compliance). Remember, however, that in certain situations a treatment may work in one patient but not in others.

The cases that follow demonstrate one example of each of the test of time and test of treatment strategies.

A father brings his 3-year-old son to see you in the GP surgery. He tells you his son has been 'off colour' and has had a fever of 38°C for the past 24 hours.

1 What avenues do you need to explore during the consultation?

A general framework for the consultation might involve considering the following:

- How well or unwell is this child – are there any features of sepsis?
- How have his symptoms evolved and what is the time course of the illness?
- Is there an obvious focus for the fever?
- Does this child have features of other serious pathology? Are red flags present?
- Should this child be referred, treated and/or reviewed?

In terms of diagnostic strategies, the first port of call should be a restricted rule-out approach or 'rule out worst case scenario', seeking to rule out serious pathology.

2 What serious pathology would you be trying to rule out?

The differential diagnosis list should include pneumonia, meningitis, appendicitis, sepsis and other causes of infection.[4] Remember, however, to think of the clinical context. In UK primary care, fewer than 1% of sick children will have a serious infection; those at highest risk of a serious infection are aged under 4 years.[5]

3 Which red flags would you ask about when seeing a febrile child?

Red flags are:

- Poor oral intake or decreased urine output (decreased frequency of wet nappies).
- Persistent listlessness, drowsiness and reduced interaction.
- A non-blanching rash, neck stiffness, photophobia, headache, and a bulging fontanelle in babies.
- Laboured breathing, wheezing or stridor.
- Continuous crying, or a weak cry in babies.
- Significant parental concern.

4 Are there any features to look for on examination that may represent 'early red flags' for meningococcal disease?

Thompson *et al.* collated the following features in a febrile child that may represent 'early red flags' for meningococcal disease:[4]

- Lethargy.
- Confusion.
- Headache.
- Leg pain leading to a reluctance to move.
- Cold hands and feet.

Note that neck stiffness is an unreliable sign in sick children: your management should not be influenced by the absence of neck stiffness if you have other significant concerns.

You establish that the child has been not been eating as much as normal but has been drinking well. He has not had any diarrhoea, vomiting or cough but has had mild coryza. He is potty trained and has passed urine as usual. His father has not noticed a rash but measured his temperature using a tympanic thermometer last night; this read 38°C. He reports his son has been able to engage in playing with toys at home but has been more tired, and he is worried that the boy may need antibiotics. The rest of the family are well.

IMPORTANT POINTS TO REMEMBER

Remember when taking histories in paediatrics to consider exploring, alongside the presenting complaint, whether the child is growing normally, whether they have had any developmental problems or problems at birth and what their immunisation history is. This is in addition to the aspects you would normally enquire about in adults (e.g. drug history, allergies, etc.). Travel history is also relevant here.

Another important point to note is that a parental perception of fever should be taken seriously, even if the parent has not measured their child's temperature. In the above case, the father used a tympanic thermometer. Tympanic and axillary thermometers are reliable in paediatrics but remember that an axillary thermometer should be used in neonates.[6]

5 How might you assess this child to help establish how unwell he is?

Your assessment will start as you talk with the father. You observe the patient as you take the history. He plays in the surgery with toys and interacts with you. His heart rate, capillary refill time and respiratory rate are within the normal range for a child of his age. He is afebrile but was last given paracetamol 2 hours previously. There is no evidence of a rash but you notice a lesion on his hand (**Figures 10.1** and **10.2**). The boy looks well hydrated and has a drink in the surgery when this is offered by his father. His chest is clear, ear, nose and throat examinations are unremarkable and his abdomen is soft and non-tender.

Note that the height of the fever is relevant to the risk of serious illness in children less than 6 months old. In this case, the child has already received paracetamol. The current advice is that antipyretics should be used if a child is in distress with a fever, and not solely to bring fever down.

6 Describe the lesion shown in Figures 10.1 and 10.2.

There is a small pink papule at the wrist on the right hand.

7 What is your differential diagnosis for this lesion?

Your differential diagnosis for such a lesion might include:

- A wart.
- Hand, foot and mouth disease (if other lesions are present).
- Chickenpox (varicella zoster – if other lesions are present).

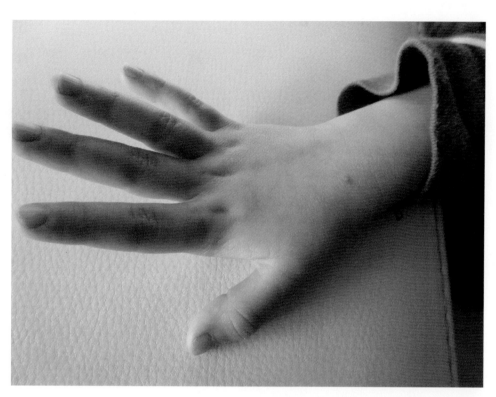

Fig. 10.1 Lesion on the right hand.

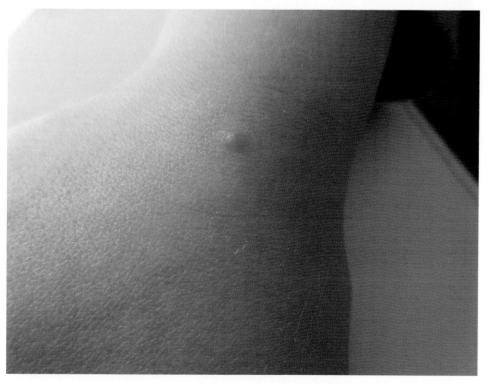

Fig. 10.2 Close-up of the lesion on the right hand.

8 What is your general impression of this child?

Given the history of fever and mild coryza, you might suspect this is a viral illness. You have not yet found any focus for the fever. Your current impression is that there are no red flags present.

9 What other investigation might you request?

You have found nothing on examination or in the history that would lead you to refer this child immediately. Consider whether you should obtain a urine sample for urinalysis and possible microscopy and culture.

CAN YOU USE THE 'TEST OF TIME' STRATEGY HERE?

The key in the above case is deciding whether the patient is potentially very unwell and needs immediate referral, whether treatment can be given in primary care or whether it is safe to 'watch and wait', given that no clear focus for the fever has been found at this early stage. Hence a thorough assessment of the child is required. It is also important to gain an impression of how well looked after and observed the child will be at home and, with appropriate safety netting, how likely the parents are to return with the child.

In the case above, the child is able to engage with you and is not drowsy or listless. His observations are in the normal range and you can find no evidence of red flags for sepsis, meningococcal disease or serious infection.

10 How would you finish the consultation with the patient's father?

To conclude, you should summarise your findings and agree a plan with his father:

- Explain that at present you cannot find a cause for the fever. It may therefore be a viral illness but you also need to rule out urinary infection.
- Explain how to manage the fever with paracetamol and ibuprofen to alleviate the distress and pain.
- Explain the importance of keeping the child well hydrated and explain how to do this.

Apply a safety net by explaining:

- Symptoms and signs that should prompt seeking further help, in particular signs of sepsis, a non-blanching rash and drowsiness, difficulty in breathing and general deterioration, including recurrent vomiting, diarrhoea, pain, high fever or features of dehydration. Make sure you fully explain the signs to look out for, such as how to check for a non-blanching rash (the glass test).
- Who they should call if they need further help.

It is wise also to advise them to return should the fever continue for more than 5 days. You could also ask the parent to check on the child during the night, and you can offer additional written information.

You elect to 'watch and wait' and use the test of time strategy.

Twenty-fours hours later the father comes back with his son. The boy has continued to have a fever but now has a widespread itchy rash. The lesion on the hand has also evolved.

11 Describe the lesion on the hand as it now appears (Figures 10.3 and 10.4).

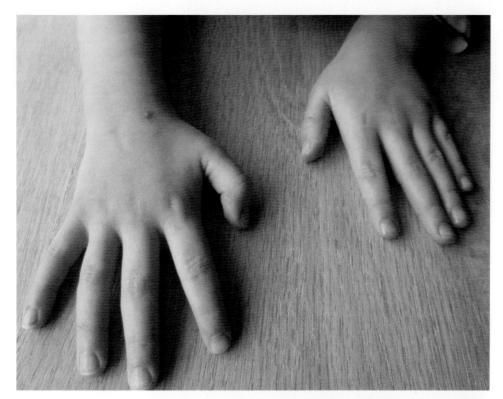

Fig. 10.3 Lesion on the right hand 24 hours later.

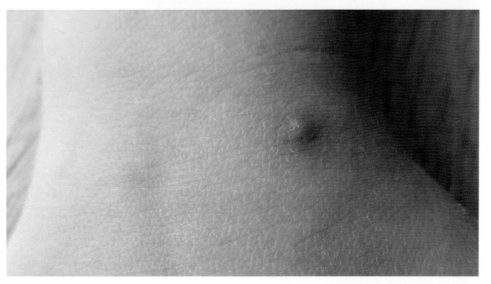

Fig. 10.4 Close-up of the lesion 24 hours later.

The lesion at the right wrist has enlarged and is now a vesicle with a pink halo.

12 You examine the rest of the patient (Figure 10.5). What is your diagnosis?

Fig. 10.5A–C
Examination of the rest of the patient.

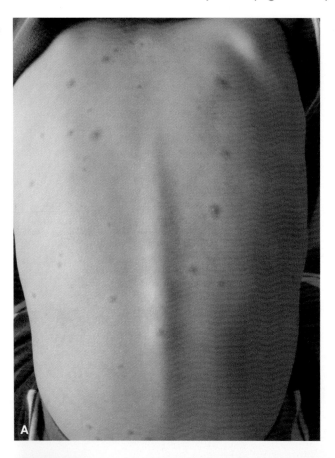

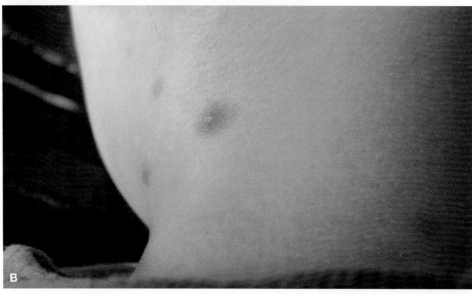

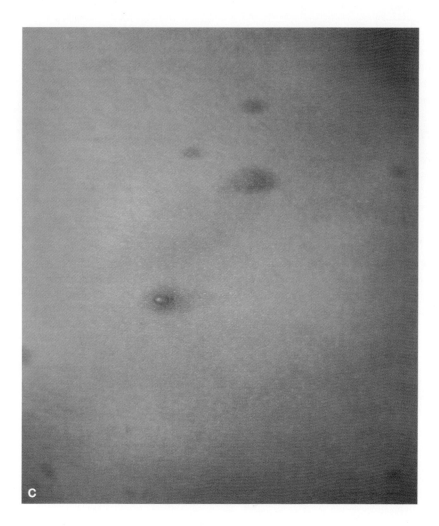

With sufficient experience of similar cases, a clinician can look at this rash and identify it as that caused by varicella zoster (chickenpox). You should check that the features of the case are consistent with this diagnosis.

In this case, crops of vesicles are accompanied by a fever of less than 40°C. The rash is itchy and has the typical features of varicella zoster (fluid-filled vesicles with a pink halo, appearing in waves over the first few days – see the details of the case above).

The parent was advised regarding the natural time course of chickenpox, and complications were mentioned as part of safety netting. These included complications such as bacterial superinfection of the spots. Note that for chickenpox, non-steroidal anti-inflammatory drugs (NSAIDs) should be avoided and paracetamol used as there is evidence to suggest that there is an increased risk of skin and soft tissue infections in children with varicella who use NSAIDs.[7]

In this case, the 'test of time' strategy worked well, based on an initial comprehensive assessment of the sick child that, as far as possible, excluded sepsis and other significant conditions.

A 35-year-old woman presents with an itchy rash on her hands. You ask the patient to tell you more about the rash. She says she noticed it about 4–6 weeks ago and is very bothered by it as it is incredibly itchy. It is localised to her hands. She has been putting moisturiser on it but wondered if she needs steroid cream as she used to have eczema as a child.

1 What further questions might you ask?

- Has she used any new products on her skin recently (skin creams, suntan lotion, detergents, etc.)?
- Does she go out to work? Does she expose her hands to any chemicals (e.g. hairdressing) or frequent handwashing (e.g. working in a kitchen)?
- Does she have any allergies and/or other medical conditions?
- Does she suffer from atopy (atopic dermatitis, asthma, allergic rhinitis)?

The patient tells you she works as a healthcare assistant. She has been using the same scented moisturiser on her hands for many years. She has not used any new products recently and has no allergies, but does suffer from mild allergic rhinitis in the summer and, as mentioned above, she used to have eczema as a child.

You examine her hands.

2 Describe the changes in the skin (Figures 10.6–10.8)

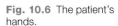 **Fig. 10.6** The patient's hands.

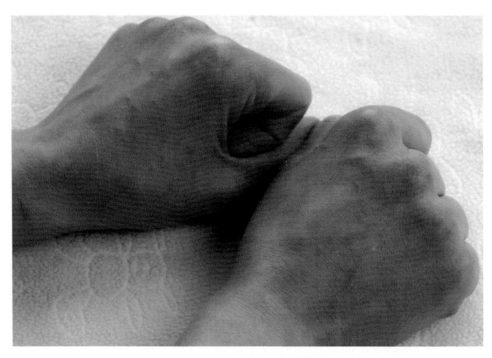

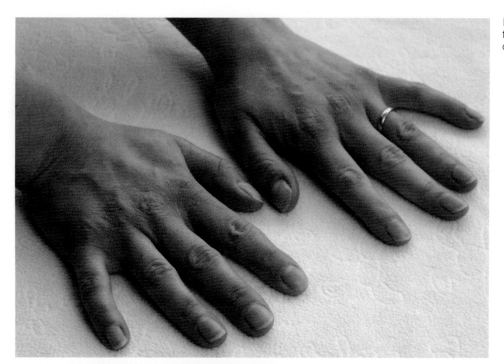

Fig. 10.7 Close-up of the skin on the dorsum of the hand.

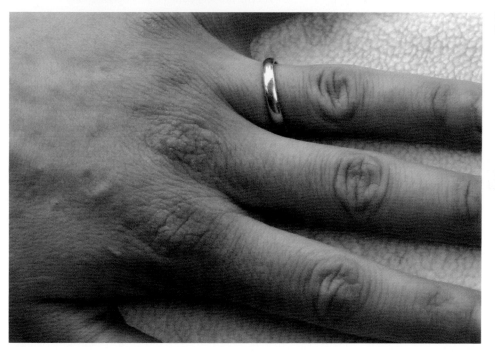

Fig. 10.8 The patient's left hand.

There is a papular rash with excoriations, erythema and scale. There is some evidence of lichen-ification and the rash is predominantly affecting the area around the finger webs (interdigital spaces) and knuckles; it is bilateral. The nails appear normal and in good condition.

Remember when looking at the skin to look for signs of infection. Itchy rashes can become infected with *Staphylococcus* after excoriation. Also look for signs of rash elsewhere. In this case, the rash is confined to the hands and is bilateral. When looking at rashes in the hands, palmar involvement is more suggestive of allergic contact dermatitis, and rashes with an asymmetrical distribution should lead you to consider fungal skin infections.

3 What does the presence of scale and lichenification indicate?

Lichenification indicates repeated rubbing or scratching of the skin. Scale and lichenification suggest this is a long-standing problem.

4 What is your differential diagnosis at this stage?

At this stage, the differential diagnosis is broad for rashes that affect the hands and includes:

- Atopic dermatitis.
- Irritant contact dermatitis.
- Allergic contact dermatitis (a type IV delayed hypersensitivity reaction).
- Pompholyx (vesicular hand dermatitis) – although in pompholyx the vesicles tend to occur on the palmar surface and sides of the fingers, which is not the case here.
- Discoid eczema, which also forms part of the differential diagnosis for a rash on the hands, but the rash here is of different morphology.
- Psoriasis: it is sometimes very difficult to distinguish between eczema and psoriasis on the hands.
- Scabies.
- Infection with gram-positive bacteria.
- Fungal infection (particularly if there is asymmetrical/unilateral involvement).

5 What risk factors for hand dermatitis does this patient have?

The patient is a healthcare professional and therefore the following may apply: contact with latex gloves, frequent handwashing and contact with chemicals such as alcohol gel.[8] Hand der-matitis is also seen more frequently in female patients and in those with a history of childhood eczema.[8]

It is important to explore in detail the nature of the person's work to identify what they are exposed to on a daily basis. You ask the patient to tell you more about her work.

The patient reports that she used to work in the outpatient department at the hospital, mainly weighing and measuring blood pressures of the arriving patients. About 8 weeks ago, she took a new role on the geratology ward. This involves much more direct contact with patients in terms of helping wash, dress and feed them. She wears gloves and washes her hands much more frequently in this role. She also uses alcohol gel frequently while at work.

6 Based on the history and clinical examination, what conclusions do you make?

The timing of the rash coinciding with the patient changing her working role to involve more frequent handwashing and the use of alcohol gel points towards an irritant contact dermatitis. She has a tendency towards atopy, which puts her at increased risk of this condition. The clinical features of the rash (symmetrical, excoriated, papular, scaly, lichenified) also fit with this diagnosis.

7 What may be causing the irritant contact dermatitis?

The patient's rash may be caused by detergents she uses in the home or at work, the scented moisturiser she is using or alcohol gel. It is likely to be exacerbated by frequent contact with water and moisture from wearing gloves.

USING THE 'TEST OF TREATMENT' STRATEGY

In the above case, the history and clinical features suggest a diagnosis of irritant contact dermatitis. We can employ the 'test of treatment' strategy by advising the following:

- Avoid using soaps and use a non-soap alternative for handwashing – this includes at work.
- Avoid the use of alcohol gel altogether if possible.
- Use emollient regularly, especially after handwashing – again this includes at work.
- To treat the very itchy areas, she could apply a moderately potent steroid such as betamethasone 0.1% ointment for 2 weeks and then use it occasionally for flare-ups.
- In order to facilitate the new routine at work, she should speak to her occupational health department about the provision of emollients and non-soap cleansers at work.

Consider organising a review in 4–6 weeks time and tell her to come back if the symptoms have not started to improve by then. Also provide a safety net for what to do should her symptoms worsen or evolve.

8 What advice might you give the patient regarding the application of corticosteroid cream and emollients?

Your advice might include the following:

- Only apply corticosteroid cream to areas affected by the rash, but use the emollient all over.
- Apply a fingertip unit of corticosteroid cream to an area the size of the hand.
- Apply creams in the direction of hair growth.
- Ideally apply the emollient first and then, if time permits, apply the corticosteroid cream 30 minutes later.[9]

In this case, the patient cut out the use of alcohol gel and used the regime detailed above. Her symptoms fully resolved.

SUMMARY

- This chapter covers 'test of time' and 'test of treatment' strategies in clinical reasoning.
- To illustrate the 'test of time' strategy, a paediatric case is described in which a boy presents with fever.
- The second case is of a patient with an itchy rash and a 'test of treatment' approach to this case is described.

REFERENCES

1   Heneghan C, Glasziou P, Thompson M, *et al.* Diagnostic strategies used in primary care. *BMJ* 2009;**338**:b946.

2   Irving G, Holden J. The time-efficiency principle: time as the key diagnostic strategy in primary care. *Fam Pract* 2013;**30**:386–9.

3   Glasziou P, Rose P, Heneghan C, Bala J. Diagnosis using "test of treatment". *BMJ* 2009;**338**:1312.

4   Thompson MJ, Harnden A, Mar CD. Excluding serious illness in feverish children in primary care: restricted rule-out method for diagnosis. *BMJ* 2009;**338**:b1187.

5   Van den Bruel A, Bartholomeeusen S, Aertgeerts B, Truyers C, Buntinx F. Serious infections in children: an incidence study in family practice. *BMC Fam Pract* 2006;**7**:23.

6   National Institute for Health and Care Excellence. Fever in under 5s: assessment and initial management. Clinical guideline [CG160]. 2013, last updated 2017. Available from https://www.nice.org.uk/guidance/cg160.

7   National Institute for Health and Care Excellence. Clinical Knowledge Summary. Bruising. 2016. Available from https://cks.nice.org.uk/bruising.

8   Perry AD, Trafeli JP. Hand dermatitis: review of etiology, diagnosis and treatment. *J Am Board Fam Med* 2009;**22**:325–30.

9   NHS. Topical corticosteroids. 2018. Available from https://www.nhs.uk/conditions/topical-steroids/.

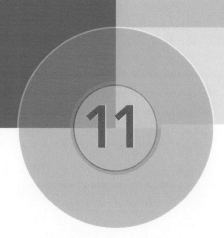

Further cases

11

INTRODUCTION

The following cases consolidate some of the themes in this book, with an emphasis on taking a full and accurate history and taking care to really 'look' when you examine a patient.

These are the hands of a 56-year-old man.

1 What observations can you make from the dorsal aspect of the patient's hands (Figures 11.1 and 11.2)?

Fig. 11.1 The patient's hands.

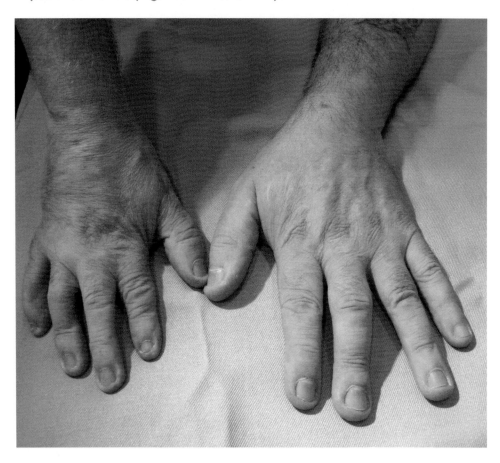

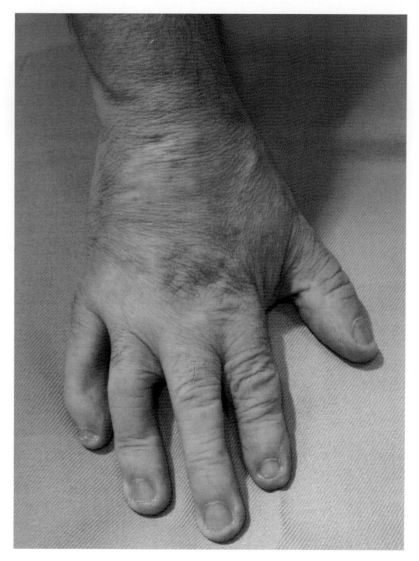

Fig. 11.2 The patient's right hand.

These are the hands of a white man. The skin and nails are in good condition. The nails are short. There is brown hair on both forearms, and a tattoo on the left forearm. The most striking observation is the discrepancy in size between the hands, the right hand being considerably smaller. The fingers and thumb on the right hand look shorter and stubbier than those on the left. The nails on the right hand are smaller. There is a small round pink lesion at the left wrist, and two linear scars on the dorsum of the left hand between the index finger and the thumb.

2 What observations can you make from observing the palmar aspect of the hands (Figures 11.3 and 11.4)?

Fig. 11.3 The palmar aspect of the hands.

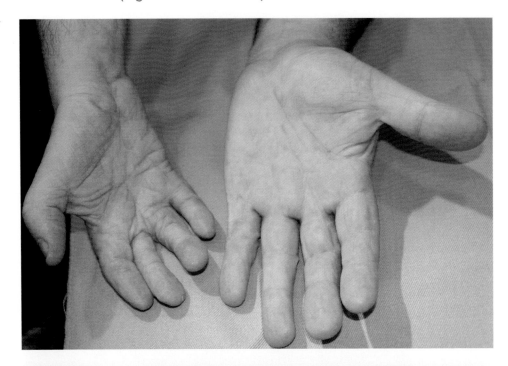

Fig. 11.4 Palmar aspect of the patient's right hand.

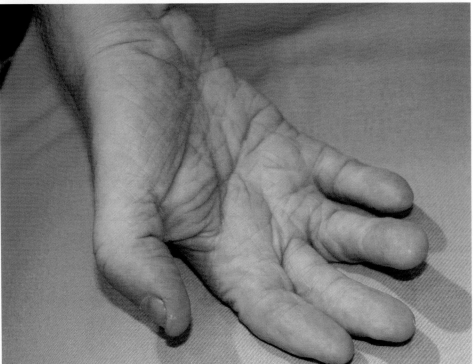

The right hand appears much smaller in size than the left hand and has a different shape. More lines are seen on the right palm than the left. There is slight webbing of the index and middle fingers amounting to minor syndactyly. There is a non-linear scar at the right wrist. The right arm looks shorter than the left arm.

3 If you were to summarise, what are the most striking features you have observed?

The most striking feature is the fact that left hand is smaller than the right, with shorter fingers and minor syndactyly. The left hand appears dysmorphic.

4 Using the 'INVITED MDC' mnemonic (see Chapter 3), which categories might you be able to use to think about possible causes for this presentation?

Category I: infection. A childhood infection such as polio is a possibility. However, the most likely category is C: congenital. A number of conditions can give rise to hypoplasia of the hand. Remember that the term 'congenital' means 'present at birth', and congenital conditions therefore either arise from a genetic problem that is inherited or occur spontaneously in the gametes, or are caused by an insult in pregnancy during embryogenesis/fetal development. In this case, the patient has a congenital condition called Poland's syndrome that has given rise to his hand anomalies.

For the majority of congenital conditions that have visible clinical manifestations, the diagnosis is made either *in utero* or in the neonatal period. This case is not about knowing the clinical features of a rare congenital condition but is described to foster skills in keen observation and to demonstrate the use of 'sieves' as an aid to diagnosis. However, we include a short note about Poland's syndrome for interest.

POLAND'S SYNDROME

Poland's syndrome is a rare (1 in 10,000 to 1 in 100,000 live births) congenital syndrome arising from an interruption in the embryonic blood supply in week 6 of gestation.[1] Specifically, the subclavian arterial blood supply is affected and becomes hypoplastic, which in turn affects the structures developing at this stage of gestation. Hence the most typical features of Poland's syndrome are unilateral aplasia or hypoplasia of the pectoralis muscle and ipsilateral hand anomalies.[1] There are associated dermatological manifestations (such as alopecia in the ipsilateral axilla), and other systemic associations have been reported.

A 68-year-old woman, who is a retired gardener, has presented to the emergency department complaining of sores on her hands. She lives with her husband and he has attended with her. She is concerned that she cannot tend to her garden properly due to painful ulcers on her hands. Her left hand was uncovered when she arrived, but her right hand was bandaged and the triage nurse has removed the dressing. Look at the photographs of the patient's hands (**Figures 11.5** and **11.6**).

Fig. 11.5 The patient's left hand.

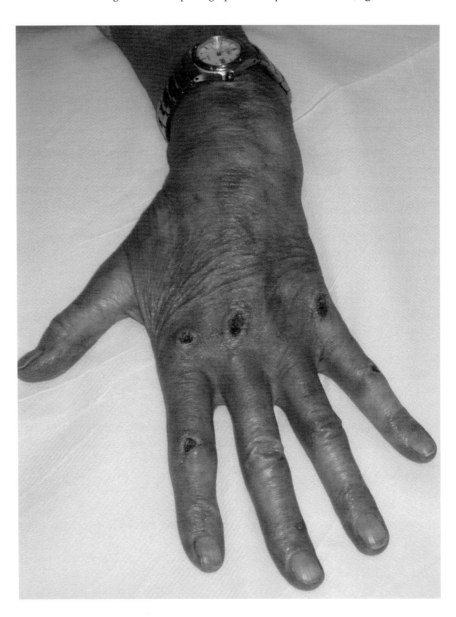

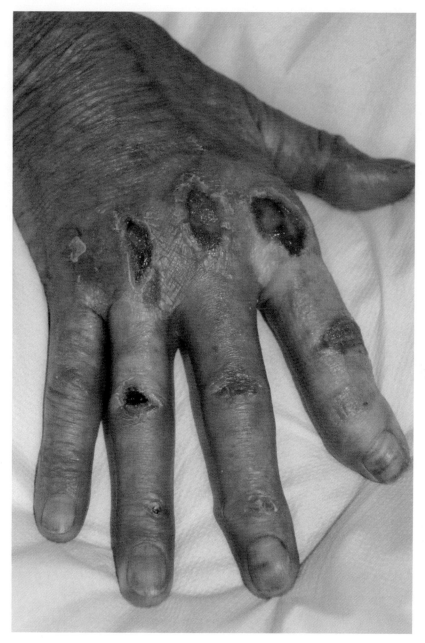

Fig. 11.6 The patient's right hand.

1 How would you describe the lesions on each hand?

The left hand has two oval-shaped lesions over the metacarpophlangeal (MCP) joints of the little and middle fingers, and one circular lesion over the MCP joint of the index finger. There are similar circular lesions over the proximal interphalangeal (PIP) joints of the index and little fingers. The lesions look like shallow ulcers that are healing. They have a pink rolled edge, are dry and have a central area of scab with no active bleeding.

The right hand has three shallow ulcers over the MCP joints of the index, middle and ring fingers, and one healed lesion over the MCP joint of the little finger. The proximal PIP joints of the index, middle and ring fingers also have similar, smaller lesions. There is erythema, oedema (as can be seen by the impression of the dressing left on the lesions at the index finger PIP joint) and yellow exudate. The lesions are in general wet, although the PIP joint lesions look drier and there are smaller, dry, healed lesions at the distal interphalangeal joints of the ring and middle fingers. There is dried exudate around the edges of the wet lesions and evidence of granulation tissue. As on the left hand, these ulcers have a pink, rolled edge.

This patient has bilateral ulcers on her hands. The ulcers on the left hand look drier than on the right hand.

2 Does a pattern recognition trigger work here?

There is no obvious pattern recognition fit here that might be a starting point for a diagnostic hypothesis.

3 What might cause bilateral ulcers on the hands?

Possible causes are:

- Exposure to chemicals.
- Infection.
- Ulcerating skin conditions that can affect the hands, such as pyoderma gangrenosum.
- Phytophotodermatitis, which can cause oozing sores.
- Neglect or abuse.
- Immunocompromise (from any cause – drugs, malignancy, HIV, etc.).
- Dermatitis artefacta.

4 Using a restricted rule-out approach, what would be on your 'must rule out' list?

Sepsis due to the open wounds is a 'must rule out'. Also, in taking a detailed history it should become clearer how these lesions came about and hence you can hopefully rule out neglect or abuse. It is also important to rule out immunodeficiency.

You review the observations taken in the emergency department. These are in the normal range. The patient reports that she feels well in herself but has presented to the emergency department because her husband had become very concerned her hands may have become infected. You take a further history from the patient.

She reports that her hands were fine until she had treatment last week for solar keratoses. She grew up in the tropics and had a lot of sun exposure. Over the last 5 years she
developed multiple solar keratoses, mainly on the dorsum of her hands. She was referred
by her GP to the dermatology department for assessment and they treated the lesions on
both hands last week. She is in otherwise good health but takes amlodipine for hypertension. She smokes 20 cigarettes per day, drinks approximately 20 units of alcohol per week
and has no known allergies. She reports that she has not had any exposure to chemicals
at home.

5 What therapies are used to treat solar keratoses?

The therapy the patient refers to could be cryotherapy, curettage, topical treatments such as
5-fluorouracil and imiquimod, or photodynamic therapy.

You ask the patient to tell you more about the treatment in the dermatology department.

The patient attended the dermatology department 4 days ago. She cannot remember the
name of the therapy but reports that she had to use a cream and then attend the department for
light therapy. On the day of the light therapy, she had both hands dressed at the dermatology
department at the end of the session. This was debilitating as she found she could not easily
smoke and do jobs around the house. Her skin looked a bit red but was otherwise fine so she
removed the dressings and sat in the garden for most of the afternoon. Over the next 72 hours
she noticed several areas becoming angry, and then sores appearing. Her husband helped her
to bandage the hands since they had started to weep but she had taken the bandages off over-
night. As it was now the weekend and her hands looked bad, her husband persuaded her to
attend the emergency department.

The history is the key to this case. Asking pertinent questions to find out exactly what hap-
pened, the time frame, what the patient did and what she noticed helps to reveal the likely
mechanism. In this case, the patient had had photodynamic therapy, which involves applying a
photosensitiser to the dorsal aspect of the hands and then exposing them to light therapy. After
the therapy, the advice is that the area is dressed for at least 48 hours to avoid further ultraviolet
exposure and hence further tissue damage. The patient did not heed this advice; the ultraviolet
exposure to her hands caused by sitting in the garden led to further tissue damage and caused
the ulcers to develop.

ON REFLECTION

In terms of diagnostic strategy for the first case, an experienced clinician who has encountered
this combination of signs before might be able to suggest a 'spot diagnosis'. We suggest that
having reviewed the pictures you consider your approach to what is most likely a novel clinical
situation. How might you set about drawing up an appropriate list of differential diagnoses?
What cognitive strategies might you employ in future possible encounters?

For the second case, on the basis of the information provided in the pictures alone, a spot
diagnosis is not possible. The key to this case is in the history. Think about how you ask patients
to 'tell you their story'. How do you seek to obtain as much information as possible about the
circumstances of the presenting complaint?

SUMMARY

- This chapter contains two cases to allow readers to consolidate their skills; these cases particularly emphasise the practising of 'careful looking' to develop visual literacy.
- The INVITED MDC mnemonic is discussed in the context of a case of congenital asymmetry of the upper limbs, with a brief description of the clinical features of this syndrome.
- The second case involves a patient who suffered burns to the hand. In this case, the restricted rule-out strategy is discussed.

REFERENCE

1   Vazirnia A, Cohen PR. Poland's syndrome: a concise review of the clinical features highlighting associated dermatologic manifestations. *Am J Clin Dermatol* 2015;**16**:295–301.

Index